Yoga

or the Art of
Transformation

WILLIAM J. FLAGG

Yoga or the Art of Transformation, W. J. Flagg
Jazzybee Verlag Jürgen Beck
86450 Altenmünster, Loschberg 9
Germany

ISBN: 9783849699529

Cover Design: © sweet_caramel - Fotolia.com

www.jazzybee-verlag.de
www.facebook.com/jazzybeeverlag
admin@jazzybee-verlag.de

CONTENTS:

PREFACE

I HAVE written this book to help myself think and now publish it to help others do so. It is, at its least, a call to thought and an aid to thinkers. With the materials I have amassed, and now put at their disposal, it would be strange if other students did not go much further than I have. To such I leave many a problem arising on the face of those materials that I have not been able to solve, and many others I have not even attempted to assail. Most of the conclusions reached have followed after the putting on paper of the facts which are their grounds, and the most important theory I have put forward is quite opposed to my former preconceptions, quite different from anything I had an idea of in the beginning.

More than a half century ago there came to my knowledge a series of strange occurrences just like those which a few years afterwards disturbed the quiet of the village of Hydesville, and which are at this time disturbing the quiet of scientific people the world over. From that time to this I have been an observer of such things and all other phenomena of occult origin. Twenty-five years ago, without having been in the meanwhile able to make anything out of them, I entered on a rather thorough course of reading in mystical literature, ancient and modern, and have continued it ever since. Fifteen years ago, baffled as much as ever, I undertook to write out some results of my observation and study, to see how they looked on paper. But it was only scant three years ago that I saw my way clear to valuable results, and later still that I decided to publish a book about them.

If the space devoted to the various religious dogmas concerning the nature and destiny of the soul should seem too large in view of the unsatisfactory outcome, it should be considered that religion having appropriated and enveloped magic — which is the real subject of the book — it had to be dug into and through in order to get at what it hid as overlying rubbish hides a treasure; and such readers as are disposed to patiently assist at the excavation will not, I fancy, waste their time; but those who think otherwise can skip two chapters (elsewhere indicated) without serious breach in the thread of the main argument. In saying "the unsatisfactory outcome", I do not mean that the soul is not worth seeking for, but only that it is not worth while to seek for it in religion — nor, in fact, anywhere else — that, our knowing apparatus being what it is, one who shall have undertaken the quest, searching for the Egyptian soul, in pyramids and caves where mummies lie, in regions of the air where hawks fly, and under the earth where Osiris holds his feasts — for the Greek soul in the stars — for the Semite soul in tombs and graves and the prison of

Allat -for the Hindu soul in the land of the fathers and land of the gods, through its series of re-births and in the bosom of Brahman — for the Mohammedan soul in Alla's hell and his prophet's paradise -for the soul of the modern spiritualist in a spiritual body and world -for souls undergoing metempsychosis, in bodies of reptiles and beasts — for the Christian soul in the raised-up and restored cadaver — will in the end be apt to remain contentedly where of old the Taoist sage, and in modern times the German one have told him he must perforce abide; namely, on the hither side of the unknowable. But if he do thorough work, in searching through religion he will have come upon magic, in searching for the secret of magic he will have found transformation, and in transformation discovered evolution.

CHAPTER I – MODERN
SPIRITUALISM ON THE SOUL

An enquiry such as this book attempts, into the nature and destiny of the soul of man, must needs begin with at least a brief review of the theories respecting it which have been offered by the various great religions of the world, of which the oldest of all, so old that it may truly be called the mother of the others, is yet so new also that we now most commonly know it by the name of "modern spiritualism".

Belief in a spiritual world contemporaneous with this natural one, and a duplicate or counterpart of it, in which, as a spirit, endowed with a body which is in like manner a duplicate or counterpart of his natural one, man goes after death, to live eternally, is as old as the world and as wide. It has been held by all primitive peoples, as it is by all savages now, whether having much other religion, or little, or none, and despite its vagueness has lived and gone along with all forms of faith, whether accepted as a dogma or not, aiding to sustain them, furnishing soil for their growth, so far as they were growths, and foundation for them to rest on, so far as they were built-up structures. It is the earliest in origin, widest in extent, most persistent in continuance, and really the best proved of all the theories ever entertained concerning the state of man after death, entertained by the learned as well as the ignorant, and whatever else the priests may have exoterically taught, or esoterically kept to themselves, has mingled with and adulterated all faiths. As believed in by primitive peoples of old and savages of modern times, by the disciples of Emanuel Swedenborg, and by all the modern spiritualists except the Kardec sect, the spiritual world is entered into immediately after death, and is man's final and eternal home, but when adopted into systematically constructed religions it has been given a subordinate place and a limited duration. Most of these consider man as having three parts, namely, a natural body that is material and perishable, a soul that is immaterial and imperishable and a shade, or form of thin matter, such as is the Karma Rupa of the Hindus, the spiritual body of the Swedenborgians and Spiritualists, the shades of the Greeks and the ghosts of all times; concerning the disposition made of these it will appear that well invented religions invest with eternal duration the soul, it alone, and never a body of any kind, whether of spirit or matter.

Probable Origin of the Belief in a Spiritual World

The facts upon which the belief in question has arisen are as real as any in nature. Nothing has been better verified by experience or more insisted on in history than the countless phenomena commonly called supernatural for which no law is known even by the wisest, and which, for that reason, modern science and philosophy have found it convenient to persistently ignore and deny, in hopes, as it were, of thereby forcing them out of belief and making them as occult as their origin and meaning have ever been. But notwithstanding scientific and philosophic simulated scorn and real ignorance, the facts are good material for the truth-seeker, and their interpretation by the common mind is as plausible, respectable and rational as could be expected, all things considered. Apparitions, sometimes of the living, sometimes of the dead, have always abundantly been seen, and never were more common than they are now. Where they were likenesses of persons dead it was easy to suppose that by the primitive men they should be taken to be the very originals they represented and as surviving after death, and the belief that they were so it is easy to suppose was the nucleus on which the belief in spirit immortality formed itself later. It is the mere spectre we are now considering, which, though a perfect likeness in face, form and movement of a living or dead person, comes without apparent purpose, and shows no meaning in expression or gesture, moving noiselessly, noticing no one, perceivable by no sense but the sight, and when accosted usually vanishing; letting stand aside for the present those others which come with an apparent purpose, as when, for instance, one is dressed in grave clothes, to signify death, or in wet ones to signify drowning, or has other accessories that tell a story, and with these others which, as if to prove themselves not merely phantasms but real presences, make themselves heard, and sometimes felt. The mere spectre seems to be without life or intelligence, very much as classic literature describes the mere shade (to which its soul had been after death temporarily united) when it was finally abandoned to endure an eternity of non-existence in Hades. In fact, it comes closely down to the natural, and closely down to the artificial too, so much so that M. D'Assier, a comtist and materialist, in his late book on "Posthumous Humanity", insists that it is not only natural but material as well, while of late other materialists have raised ghosts by artificial means, which they claim to be as good as any, and fondly think in doing so they have exploded supernaturalism forever. That in the minds of primitive men even such stupid shadows could induce a belief in a world of spirits is not hard to think; it would be hard to think otherwise. To such the conclusion must have been irresistible that forms so clearly shown to the sight must be discernible by the other senses also, and have life, thought and feeling like the once living, thinking and feeling men they stood for;

that beings thus supposed, who came and went, and came and went again, must come from and go to a somewhere of which they were habitual residents, and which somewhere might be in the skies that daily and hourly exhibited to those primitive minds even more wonderful things, or in the earth, also full of wonders, now heaving and shuddering in earthquakes and now spouting fire in volcanoes, in any case a region out of reach of man's powers of exploration. Such a belief, once induced, no matter how arising — whether in the way supposed or some other does not affect the argument — this most important consequence must have followed: thenceforth all messages to men from the occult powers, supposing such to be, and to send messages, must needs conform to it or go unheeded ; especially must conform to it such as related to the loved and mourned for dead. And just as pent-up waters escaping from the dam that held them must follow the course of the first little rill that finds a way over its crest, deepening and widening its channel as they flow, so did ghost and ghost-land belief, however slender its beginning, in time make place for itself in human belief. This but states a principle governing all teaching, namely, that it must be fitted to the receptivity of those who are to be taught. Respect must be had to their beliefs and unbeliefs, knowledge and ignorance, their religion, morality, superstitions and prejudices, only disturbing these so far as is necessary to convey the intended instruction. Just as molten metal has to submit to whatever limitations the mould it is poured into imposes, revelations, to gain reception have to adapt themselves to receptivities. It is the same even with discoveries men make in material nature provable to the senses; if they come out of time they have to bide their time for acceptance into scientific belief. In view of this Moses was right when he gave the Jews a cosmogony which they could, in their intellectual condition, understand, and a morality not too good for them to live up to, although as priest of Egypt he must have been learned in all that was taught to Solon and Pythagoras, and known a morality as high and pure as theirs.

Father Abraham, always ready to receive his god Jehovah, certainly would never have allowed himself to be dictated to by Osiris or Bel. The apparition in the conventional form of Bacchus which gave the warning that saved Alexander's army from being destroyed in a night would have failed of its mission had it personated one of the gods of the enemy. So, too, when the city of Aphutus, being besieged by King Lysander, was saved by a dream sent to him by Jupiter Ammon, as he believed, in obedience to which he raised the siege and rapidly retreated, the King heeded the warning because it came from a deity he was acquainted with. Especially is it requisite that the accepted cosmogony of the times be humored. The scriptures of the Jews humored theirs, a poor one it is true, but the only one they had. To them the earth remained fixed and the heavens moved round it, and Jehovah let them have it so, although he must have known better, since the Book of Job, truly rendered, says he himself "hung the earth in its sockets". Had the fair spirit of the Spring of Lourdes made herself apparent to the little girl with sore eyes as her grandmother, the chapel that has since arisen there, begemmed with gifts from thousands of pilgrims whom the waters have healed, would not be seen to-day, but in its stead an iron fence and a policeman, such as the priests did, in fact, cause to be placed there, from fear that anything miraculous would in modern France only bring ridicule upon them, until its good-for-naught of an Emperor Napoleon III by decree made them let the thing go on. The Spirit, therefore, wisely gave as her name, when under direction of her priest the child asked for it, as "the Immaculate Conception", a droll phrase to make a name of, to be sure, but a popular catchword with good Catholics just then when the Church had woke up to the importance of the question how the maternal grandmother of Jesus came by her baby. The beautiful, if improper, Aspasia, threatened with serious disfigurement by a growth upon her face, prayed to Venus to heal it, in response to which the goddess came in person and prescribed an unction to be made by pulverizing a dried rose from a chaplet then hanging on her image in the temple, which being done not only cured, but made her more beautiful then ever. But whether a goddess Venus ever ruled in earth or heaven remained as doubtful afterward as before. In fact, if we view these two last-named spirits as objective realities, it is conceivable that the ancient Goddess of Love and the modern Lady of the Spring were one and the same being. The Hindus make their god Siva say, pray to whatever god you please, I will answer your prayer, which is recognizing diversity of receptivities and acknowledging the necessity of recognizing them, and at the same time proving Great Siva to be high above jealousy and an example to some other gods we wit of.

And so the idea of a world of spirits peopled by the dead having once got hold on the minds of men, after that the entire body of mystical revelation must necessarily ratify and confirm it.

We have been considering the effect of the mere spectre on the simple minds of primitive men in causing them to believe in a world of spirits, a result which might not have happened to instructed minds, but when those occult powers which manifest an interest in human affairs by messages of instruction, warning and guidance, adapting their modes of communication to that primitive belief, and, so to say, taking advantage of it, spoke by the mouths of the spectres, put meaning into their eyes and expression into their actions, and through them predicted truly the future, prescribed medicines that cured, and gave comfort to the bereaved, not only the simple, but the instructed must be excused if they believed. Instances to illustrate this are common today. Intelligent men who, like the body of educated people of European race during the last two centuries, have ignored all such manifestations of the occult, not deigning to honor them so far as to disbelieve them, when at length confronted with the facts in a way that compels belief are apt to accept not only the facts themselves, but the interpretation which believers in them had commonly put upon them, namely, that they prove a spiritual immortality. And such of them as have rejected religion on the ground that its origin was in the supernatural only and the supernatural impossible, as soon as they come to believe in the supernatural at all, will be apt to run and join the nearest church. Three college-bred men, all of them confirmed skeptics, all near sixty years of age, and, as veteran lawyers, experienced in examining proofs, one a brilliant orator and ex-governor, one a brilliant editor, an author and ex-judge, and the other a brilliant conversationalist, attended together, some twelve years ago, a series of séances held by Mrs. Hollis-Billing which had the effect to convince them that the supernatural was possible. Thus far one identical series of observed facts brought three men to one and the same conclusion. And what next? One, who had been bred in the Catholic Church, returned again to her bosom, and ten years later died happy in her communion and faith; one, whose wife happened to be an old-school Presbyterian, incontinently went and entered into that communion, became one of its shining lights, and died in it; while the other relapsed into his original skepticism and died an unbeliever.

CHAPTER II - HINDU SOULS

In its essential nature Hinduism is beyond question the best, greatest and most admirable religious and philosophical system in the world. Its beginning was too early for its age to be computed, and, unlike all the other great religions of antiquity, it has endured down to the present time, and is in full life to-day. Its votaries, because largely restrained by its beneficent teachings from engaging in wars, whose attendants are forever pestilence and famine, and of the doctrine, inherited from still more early ancestor worship, that many sons are advantageous to the dead father of them, have multiplied by hundreds of millions on the soil of India while its offshoot. Buddhism, has spread over and now covers with other hundreds of millions, the larger and more enlightened parts of Asia, all of them holding steadfast to the faith of their fathers, despite the persuasions of Christian missionaries, however earnest or well backed by ships of war. And there can be no better proof that Hinduism is in full life to-day than the fact that pious Hindus are actually turning the tables on us, by sending hither learned and eloquent teachers to convert their would-be converters, teachers whom many of our learned men listen to with attention and profit, because they have indeed something to tell.

Hinduism rests on a body of scriptures of varying degrees of authority. Of these the Upanishads, a part of the Vedas, are firmly believed to be divine revelations, to which even the highest philosophy must conform, and the best work done in the less authoritative writings of saints and sages has been in efforts to reconcile them with reason and with each other. Of the Upanishads Max Müller in his Vedanta Philosophy, p. 23, says : "The impression they leave on the mind is that they are sudden intuitions or inspirations, which sprang up here and there and were collected afterwards, and yet there is system in all these dreams, there is background to all these visions. There is even an abundance of technical terms used by different speakers so exactly in the same sense that one feels certain that behind all these flashes of religious and philosophical thought there is a distant past, a dark background of which we shall never know the beginning". The same good authority tells us that etymologically the word Upanishad means "sitting near a person", which cannot but remind us that the French word séance has been adopted to designate attendance at a modern spiritualistic circle and must favor the belief that these Hindu scriptures were revelations made to circles of ancestor worshippers of old, by automatic writing, trance speaking, etc., just as mediumistic "communications" are made to us now. It is also worthy of note, that like most such communications, the Upanishads are quite undevotional. Says Müller, page 16 of the same work: "These Upanishads are philosophical treatises, and their fundamental principle might seem with us to be subversive of all religion. In these Upanishads the whole ritual and sacrificial system of the Veda is not only ignored, but directly rejected as useless, nay, mischievous. The ancient gods of the Veda are no longer recognized. And yet these Upanishads are looked upon as perfectly orthodox, nay, as the highest consummation of the Brahmanic religion". On page 113 we read that most of Buddha's doctrines were really those of the Upanishads. There is no esoteric aspect to Hinduism. Excepting the lowest caste, who would hardly care for or be able to appropriate its higher teaching, all are free to draw from the abundant sources of its wisdom supplied by the sacred writings or the oral instructions of living sages, as much as they are mentally and morally fit to receive, and as fast as they become so fit. Symbols, idols and even the gods above are merely aids to thought and contemplation, and devotional worship of them but an introductory discipline for preparing the worshipper to do without them. The more a Hindu knows of his religion the less devout he is; the perfected Yogi does not pray at all, he only meditates on what he wants and it comes to him. But it is a graded religion, wherein each grade of intelligence can find its fitting temple there to remain, content with the comfort it affords him, or going up higher when worship there has developed him beyond its power to satisfy him. A Hindu may attend on temple gods perhaps for ten years, and then having by that means rendered himself so spiritual as not to need them, abandon them forever. " This was brought about, " says Müller, page 16, " by the recognition of a very simple fact which nearly all other religions seem to have ignored. It was recognized in India from very early times that the religion of a man cannot be and ought not to be the same as that of a child ; and again that the religious ideas of an old man must differ from those of an active man of the world". From such a system toleration necessarily flowed. Hinduism punishes no man for his religious faith.

In the Bhagavadgita the Supreme Spirit says as generously as Siva, lately quoted, "even those who worship idols, worship me".

God

Consistent with the foregoing is the instituting of two Brahmans, the one, an impersonal principle, exalted by negation of attributes quite out of sight, an It and not a He ; the other, masculine and personal, invested with all divine qualities and actively engaged in ruling the world. The higher god is found in only well elaborated religions; the lower is found in every religion. Zeus, the Egyptian Osiris, the Assyrian Bel, the Phoenician Bacchus and the Jewish Jehovah were of these latter.

The Cosmos

The impersonal Brahman creates the Universe by breathing it out, and again destroys it by breathing it in, both the creation and destruction being periodical. This may be called the real Universe, which is Brahman itself, and not merely pervaded by it. The Universe, as man knows it, is the creature of man's avidya, Nescience, Ignorance; in fact, his knowledge of things consist in his ignorance of them, each one's individual ignorance being helped by the erroneous thought of the race collectively, amounting to something like a cosmic force. Which suggests Berkeley's statement that each one of us perceives as really existing what does not exist, not merely by force of his own thinking so, but by the aid also of the concentrated thought of all mankind.

The Origin of Man

Every religion has a different account to give of the reasons which moved its creative god to make man, as well as of the way in which he did it. As to the reason that prevailed with the Hindu creator, " we are told that Pragapate (Visva) stood alone in the beginning, that he had no happiness when alone, and that meditating on himself he created many creatures. He looked on them and saw they were like stone, without understanding, and standing about like lifeless posts. He had no happiness, and thought that he would enter into them that they might awake". Thus it may be said that man was made that God might be happy. As to the way it was done, in the Upanishad treating of it various details are given, which are, however, included in the following general statement, same page: "O Saint, this body is without intelligence, like a cart. By whom has this body been made intelligent, and who is the driver of it? Then Pragapate answers that it is He who is standing above, passionless amid the objects of the world, endless, imperishable, unborn and independent; that it is Brahman that made this body intelligent, and is the driver of it". It is the higher Brahman which does this, of which man is, so to speak, the manifoldness.

Nature of the Soul

According to Hindu belief, the soul is "neither our body nor our minds, not even our thoughts, of which most philosophers are so proud, but all of these are conditions merely to which it has to submit, as fetters by which it is chained, nay, as clouds by which it is darkened, so as to lose the sense of its substantial oneness with God".

Soul is Brahman and Brahman is soul. Soul has but three qualities — it is, it perceives and it enjoys. But the word "Atman", commonly translated soul, is better rendered as Self, whether regarded in its divine or human aspect, by knowing which we are more helped to a comprehension of what in our terminology must still be called, for want of a better phrase, the union of the soul with God, than we could be by a whole chapter of explanation. The importance of this distinction is made to appear by the following passages from the Upanishads :

"In the beginning there was Self" ; "He, therefore, who knows the Self, after having become quiet, subdued, satisfied, patient and collected, sees self in Self, sees all as Self" ; "The Self, smaller than small, greater than great, is hidden in the heart of the creature" ; " Verily a husband is not dear that you may love the husband, but that you may love the Self, therefore the husband is dear".

Earthly Life an Evil

Like all civilized peoples, except our three Jewish sects of Jews, Christians and Mohammedans, the Hindus believe undoubtingly that the life of man on earth consists of a succession of lives of one soul in many bodies, lives which are not blessings but curses, and will continue to succeed each other.in a vicious round that must be unending while the world lasts, unless the sufferer, by a resolute renunciation of the will to live, and yoga practice soon to be described, can slip out of it and by a short path get into the bosom of Brahman.

The Land of the Fathers

As a place of demure for the Hindu soul between reincarnations a portion of the old spiritual world of Vedic hymns is appropriated. It is called "the land of the fathers", and is reached by "the pathway of the fathers", which means a life of good works, charitable or devotional. There it is that clothed in the "subtle bodies" they wore under their fleshly ones souls enjoy refuge from the ills of earth life until they have exhausted the stock of acquired merit that gave them admission, after which they must return to earth, enter new bodies and undergo renewed tribulation. It is while tarrying in this paradise that they receive the devotional offerings of their surviving descendants, in the form of sacrifices and feasts, and which they repay with guardian counsel and care.

The land of the fathers corresponds to the spiritual world of Swedenborg and modern spiritualism, as the "subtle body" temporarily worn as above does to the spiritual body in which, according to these the unreturning soul exists eternally, and as it is presumable it was believed to do by the primitive Hindus while yet ancestor worship was their only religion.

The Land of the Gods

This is a higher paradise than the other, which mere good works will not win, appropriated to ascetics who have gone so far on the way to final deliverance from all life as to have become unfitted for earthly life. In the land of the gods, the subtle body is still worn. This is not cast aside until final enfranchisement from all embodiment is obtained, which can be done without return to earth, for it seems yoga can be practiced in the land of the gods as well as here below.

Karma

The doctrine of Karma, or the subjection of the soul in a given earth life to conditions having a punitive, disciplinary and compensatory relation to its conditions and actions in a former one is something superadded to the doctrine of re-incarnation and not necessarily connected with it. Hindu teachers present it as resulting by the automatic working of the law of cause and effect, whereby, without calling in the aid of a presiding deity, sin committed in one life necessarily causes a corresponding punishment in another, error in one brings about its own correction in another, and hardship in one induces compensating advantage in another. As Plotinus states the same principle in the Enneads, ii. 474: "The divine law is inevitable and has the power to carry its judgment into effect". But by divine law he means, as he writes in the Enneads, ii. 291, the law of nature. No acknowledged facts prove this Karma doctrine to be true. It is usually defended by appeal to some law of compensation by which human conditions which are so unequal, when viewed within the range of a single life, are intended to be averaged up, so that conditions of wealth and poverty, health and sickness, grandeur and abasement shall be equalized, and the dealings of God with man justified. But the doctrine is defective and inconsistent with itself; to minds of the common sort this gloss put upon it to make it presentable can hardly bring conviction. It is easier to see in it a convenient and most effective priestly device for keeping the vulgar in order, and to understand how, that being so, it was set up as a religious dogma, than to find for it any scientific basis.

16

Yoga in Hinduism

Like our own word religion, taken in its original sense, yoga means junction, but to the Hindu believer it means more than to any other, signifying nothing less than this, that having always been Brahman, a man, by means of certain practices, comes to know it — that's all. For a soul to become God is more than is compassed by the word in its simple sense, but it is less than a Hindu means when he pronounces it. For it to be absorbed in God is still less. For a soul, by works of grace or other means, to raise itself to the level of God, and be united to Him in whatever way conceivable, is still less. Yoga makes the soul to know that from eternity unto eternity it is God, that, as Sankara states it, "it has become God by being God". The process by which one attains to the knowledge that makes him consciously Brahman will be given at length later on. For the present, it is enough to say that it consists in renouncing the will to live, and all earthly allurements and interests, and in solitude and quietude holding the mind to meditations such as will best oncentrate it, and thereby reduce the flow of thought to the least possible point, so that, in the language of a Hindu sage, the man "is as it were delivered from his mind". Yoga may be practiced either with or without devotion. The manuals of Yoga are mostly made up from the Upanishads, which are philosophical and magical, rather than religious works. The priest is not called in nor the temple resorted to. Alone in the forest, the seeker after enfranchisement goes through mental and physical exercises that have their beginning and end within his own body and mind. Postures are carefully taken, but kneeling is not one of them. The eyes are turned in this direction and that, but not to heaven, not higher than the forehead or the top of the brain. Word formulas are repeated, but they are not prayers. In his early religious life, perhaps, the recluse has concentrated his mind on God Siva in the sky or his image in the temple, but now he directs it to this and that part of his own body, or on some one point of fact or thought or thing, or on simple vacuity, the best of all.

The doctrine is that Yoga operates the perfecting of the body, and such perfecting Plotinus no doubt had in mind when, in the Enneads, ii. 298, he wrote: "If each body were as perfect as the Universe is, it would be completely sufficient unto itself. It would have no danger to fear, and the soul which is present in it, instead of being present there, could communicate life to it without quitting the intelligible world".

And being thus an affair of the body, in bodily life alone, either physical or spiritual, must yoga work be done. But the striving and waiting that is to lead the soul out of the darkness that hides it from itself into the light that reveals its eternal godship may not accomplish its end in one life, nor perhaps in more than one. Time is required for all the operations of nature, and yoga is a natural operation. As it goes on certain miraculous powers are developed, but the true yogi seldom exerts them. To him they are like flowers by the wayside to one who hastens on a long journey. They tell him the end is near, but the gathering of them would hinder him in reaching it. The enfranchisement, when at last it is gained, finds the soul still bound to a body, and then there is a being "whose feet", in the words of Plotinus, "touch the earth while his head lifts itself above the sky", and this consciously.

Of such beings wonderful stories are told and believed in India, for they are there held to be more than demi-gods. They determine the duration of their own lives as men, and sometimes indefinitely extend them. Sometimes they largely influence the affairs of men, sometimes they bodily vanish and sometimes drop the body in death, as unenfranchised souls do. And though thus becoming completely rid of the flesh, some have, after long lapses of time, voluntarily and consciously re-embodied themselves and returned as messiahs to endure humanity for the good of humanity.

The points of difference between the great sect of Buddhism, with its 400 millions of followers and its parent Hinduism, though in many respects they are important, are still not so for the purposes of this our enquiry, but the following statement of a Buddhist of the Ceylon school, found in the "Buddhist Catechism" of Subhadra Bikshu, S. 150, is well worth quoting:

Question : " What is the main difference between the doctrine of Buddha and other religions ?"

Answer: "Buddhism teaches the highest kindliness and wisdom without a personal God; the highest understanding without revelation; a moral order of the world and just compensation which are of necessity consummated on the principle of the laws of nature and of our own being; a continuity of individuality without an immortal soul ; an eternal beatitude without a local heaven ; a possibility of redemption without a vicarious redeemer; a salvation at which each one is his own savior, and which can be attained by one's own strength, and already gained in this life and upon this earth without prayer, sacrifice, penance, and outward rites, without consecrated priests, without the mediation of saints, and without the action of divine grace " — namely, by the practice of Yoga.

CHAPTER III - EGYPTIAN SOULS

The Egyptian religion is a dead one, and considering how many thousand years it prevailed it is not strange that accounts given of it should vary and conflict, even those afforded by its own records and monuments. In a book of uncertain age and origin, but for which great antiquity and authority is claimed, entitled "The Virgin of the World" by "Hermes Trismegistus", we read that God formed out of a certain something to which the name of "self-consciousness" is given, "myriads of souls" and "traced the limits of their sojourn on the heights of nature, so that they might turn the wheel according to the laws of order and of their wise discretion, for the joy of their father", and commanded them thus: "Quit not the place assigned to you by my will. The abode which awaits you is Heaven, with its galaxy of stars and its thrones of virtue. If you attempt any transgression against my decree, I swear by my sacred breath, by that elixir of which I formed you, and by my creative hands, that I will speedily forge for you chains and cast you into punishment". And then he formed living beings of human shape (living and procreating, but without souls). Then he gave the rest of his stuff to the loftiest souls, inhabiting the region of the gods in the neighborhood of the stars, being those just named, saying: "Work, my children, offspring of my nature, take the residue of my task, and let each one of you make beings in his image. I will give you the models".

The souls thus commanded set to work and created the different races of animals below the degree of man; and thereupon became proud of their skill, and in their pride disregarded the command to remain where they were placed and "moved about ceaselessly"; for which offense God punished them by imprisoning them in human organisms, a proceeding so much against their wills, we are told, that when they learned their sentence "they were seized with horror". Some sighed and lamented, as when some wild, free animal is suddenly enchained; some hissed like serpents, or gave vent to piercing cries. "Must we quit", they exclaimed, "these vast effulgent spaces, this sacred sphere, all these splendors of the Empyrean and of the Happy Republic of the gods, to be precipitated into those vile and miserable abodes?" Thus Egyptian wisdom made the fall of man to occur before he was born, and sinning souls to come to their punishment at birth instead of going to it at death.

Many Christian writers give out that the Egyptians believed in a resurrection of the body, arguing that otherwise they would not have built such costly tombs nor so carefully embalmed corpses to be held in them.

For want of other reason, especially for the embalmment, it is insisted that it must have been believed that the mummies were to arise and again receive their souls. But there is nothing in Egyptian learning to prove this; on the contrary, we find there three other distinct reasons for embalming, either of which is good and sufficient to exclude the need of the supposition of any resurrection, if not to show the necessity of the practice itself.

The first reason was that it was to save the elements, held to be gods, from pollution. The book just quoted from tells us that when mankind began to die and dead bodies to abound, the four elements appeared before God the Creator, and each in turn protested against being made the receptacle of corpses. Earth objected to burial, fire to cremation, water to having its purity defiled by decaying matter, and air to being tainted by effluvia from the unburied. In consequence of these embarrassing appeals Osiris and Isis were sent to earth, who taught men the art of mummifying. (So says this book, but Maspero, as we shall see, makes the instruction come from the god Anubis, master of sepulture).

Here was a most proper sanitary measure veiled by fable. The second reason was that the preserved corpses, like the Buddhist and Christian relics, were supposed to be effective in invoking the soul that had left it. The third, probably an afterthought, was that a soul thus at call must be excused from attendance before the high court of the dead, and from undergoing punishment decreed by it while the mummy lasted. A fourth and less well-considered reason was that unless the soul be held to attendance on the body it would be liable to enter into those of beasts and half-decayed astral "shells".

Professor Rawlinson, in his "Religions of the Ancient World", asserts that embalmment was for the purpose of keeping the body in good order to receive back its soul again in a subsequent re-incarnation, of which there was to be a long series ending at last in re-absorption in the supreme being. But he cannot be right. The Egyptians had too much brains to suppose a body without any in its cranium could serve as living receptacle of a returning soul, which could always find new-born babes to enter into without needing to rob the tomb. Again, that industrious Egyptologist, Gerald Massey, declares that the mummy once swaddled and coffined never walked again; and Herodotus, who in the days of embalment went to Egypt, studied the process, and learned of the beliefs then and there prevailing, says simply that the soul of the departed returned to earth and entered the body of a man. But there is yet another supposition.

The contradictions in the accounts we have of the religious beliefs of Egypt are no doubt mostly due to the enormous length of her history, though In the light of recent discoveries many accounts must be now wholly discredited. Then again, she had a migratory capital, each movement of which from the delta of the Nile upward towards its cataracts involved a change of gods and a modification of the worship of them. In the confusion thus arising the late work of M. Maspero on "The Ancient History of Oriental Peoples", and which gives the latest news from the explorations, brings welcome light, and by aid of it, in connection with what was before known, the natural history of the Egyptian soul may be clearly enough traced for present purposes. We now at last find the true rationale of the mummy and its pyramid. The key to their mystery and to Egypt's whole religious system is seen to be a dogma, originating in very early and savage times, which, though so arising, like others of equally low origin, has by virtue of that strange principle prevailing in all religions which makes a dogma seem true in proportion as the time is long, which removes its grounds and sanctions from reach of scrutiny, persisted through all stages of subsequent enlightenment, making even that enlightenment subservient to it, while in return rendering it of small avail for good. The dogma in question made the immortality of the soul depend on the preservation of the body, quite the opposite of the Christian fundamental belief that the soul confers immortality on the body, or at least will do so when the world comes to an end. Long before mummies were embalmed or pyramids built, the inhabitants of the Nile Delta in some way adopted this notion, first proclaimed, may be, by some naked worker of magic spells, the equal in wisdom of our red-skinned medicine-men, or a black-skinned mumbo-jumbo man, and fortuitously taking root in the minds of a tribe of other naked people even more ignorant than he, afterwards, as centuries rolled on, to be consecrated by the developed intelligence of a civilized and great nation as infallible truth.

As a result the Egyptians very early selected for the interment of their dead rocky or sandy, rather than low and moist soils, because in dry ground bodies would keep longer and souls survive longer; which custom continued even after the god Anubis, master of sepulture, came and taught men the art of embalming as a better method of ensuring eternal life. But before the coming of the undertaker god, and even after considerable progress had been made in civilization, no better home for the soul (or what stood for it) was provided than the grave in dry sands or tomb among the rocks, where it had to lie with its body and live with it as best it could. In the more developed psychology of Egyptian sages the man was composed of a material body, a double of it in thin ghostly stuff, and a soul so far incorporeal that it could only manifest itself by taking the form of a hawk, in which to come and go and visit its body in its dire abode, though without ever entering either it or its double, either in life or death. But in the beginning this, the true soul, played no part. The survivor at death was the mere double. This was supposed, as it has everywhere been by those who have conceived it, including Swedenborg and modern spiritualists also, to be a duplicate of its late incasement, like it needing food, drink and raiment, so that there was danger notwithstanding its quasi immortality and the fact that its man had already died once, the poor thing in its gloomy hole would die of starvation, a fear confirmed by the common belief that famishing ghosts did actually come forth in the night season to prowl and plunder and even, as vampires, suck the blood of those who slept. It was to prevent this night walking that the custom arose (of awful consequence to the human race) of burying with the dead at the first interment, and from time to time afterwards depositing within their reach supplies of food and drink and other comforts, which served not only to purchase exemption from such depredations, but secured to the givers the good will and friendly offices of the doubles, whatever that might count for. Thus the universal and long consecrated custom of feeding the dead is seen to have originated in fear, howbeit, since it was their surviving relatives on whom the duty devolved, it was natural that love would soon or late take the place of fear as motive or at least mingle with it.

Concerning the kind of existence the double was supposed to lead so interred with its body, whether in grave or tomb, Maspero says: "It there retained its character and its figure as above ground; double before the funeral, it remained double afterwards, with ability to accomplish in its way all the functions of animal life. It moved, went and came, breathed, spoke, received the homage of devotees, but without joy and like a machine, more by reason of an instinctive horror of annihilation than from any real love of life. Regret for the daylight world it had quitted troubled incessantly its inert and gloomy existence". And he quotes from a tablet as late as the time of the Ptolemies a lament supposed to be uttered by a double in its tomb:

"O, my brother, cease not to eat and drink, get drunk and make love. Give yourself up to your desires night and day and while you can live grieve for nothing. .... Here is a land of slumber and darkness, a place where the inhabitants sleep in their mummied forms never more to awake, never more to behold their brothers, fathers, mothers, oblivious of their wives and children O, give me to drink of running water Set my face to the wind from the north and my feet on the river's shore that refreshing breezes may kiss away my grief".

On the other hand, the following is the discourse a living man is supposed to have held with his soul, copied from a papyrus now at Berlin:

"I say to myself every day: What returning health is to one who has been ill and rises from his bed of suffering to go out into the open court, such is death. I say to myself every day : Like breathing there the perfumed air, seated in the pleasant shade of an extended curtain, such is death. I say to myself every day: Like sitting on a flower bank in the land of drunkenness, breathing sweet odors, such is death. I say to myself every day: Like an inundating flood, like a warrior in combat, whom none can withstand, such is death. I say to myself every day: Like a clearing sky, like a hunter who, following his game too far, suddenly finds himself in a country he knows nothing of, such is death".

The conflict between the two statements cannot be reconciled by the one being uttered by a double and the other by a living man concerning his soul, for there is no reason for supposing there was ever a belief that the soul could be happy and the double miserable, but must, like innumerable other conflicting statements which the stones and manuscripts of Egypt make, be attributed to their relating to different times and places during the enormously long course of Egypt's history, in which the seat of government was many times changed, and with it the presiding deity, followed by modifications in worship and creed or to their representing beliefs accepted by different grades of mind. There was abundant room in time and space and in the range of intelligence from high to low to admit any conceivable number of diverse beliefs concerning what must ever lie outside of knowledge. A gradual improvement continued to go on, but to the last the soul proper was but a mere visitor to the tomb of its mummy, of which the double was, on the other hand, the constant companion — a thing of bodily needs, that must be fed and comforted, if not always by real food and drink, etc., then by representation of these in sculpture and painting.

But if dead men were troublesome to the living, dead gods were much more so, to both the living and the dead. In contriving their anthropomorphic deities the Egyptian theologians were logical enough to make them mortal. They could die of disease, or age, though not so early in life as men, and could even be murdered as Osiris was. And since their doubles too derived immortality from their bodies, gods had to be as carefully buried or entombed. At first cemeteries were established for them on mountain slopes, and one of the most ancient titles given the defunct deities was "those who are on the sands", but when embalming was discovered they had the benefit of it. "Every Nome", says Maspero, "had the mummy and the tomb of its dead god, mummy and tomb of Anhouri at Thenis, mummy of Osiris at Mendes, mummy of Tourmou at Heliopolis. Many would not admit that their names were changed in changing their mode of existence: Osiris defunct remained Osiris still, Nit or Hathor remained Nit or Hathor at Sais or at Dendera, but Phtah of Memphis became Sokaris when he died, etc". And in the other life their doubles fared no better than men as to hunger, thirst and gloom, though their ennui was somewhat beguiled by their being allowed to exercise the functions of rulers over them who in life had owed them fealty, the same as before. Nevertheless, their dispositions were sadly altered for the worse. Gods who while they lived were distinguished for goodness, once they found themselves in the tomb, became tyrannical, rapacious and ferocious. A mortal summoned before Osiris even, in his youth so loving and kind, came, as is related, "in fear and trembling, and none among gods or men dare look him (Osiris) in the face, and the great and small are alike to him. He spares none because they love him. He carries off the infant from its mother and the old man who crosses his path; all beings, filled with fear, implore before him, but he turns not his face towards them". "Neither the living nor the dead could escape his fury except on condition of constantly paying tribute to and feeding him like a simple human double". Gifts intended for the double of one who owed fealty to a dead god must pass through his hands and he was sure to deduct for his own use a round commission before he delivered them.

M. Maspero could not be expected to tell his readers about any esoteric religion held in secret by the priests, or imparted to those only who were intelligent enough to reject the exoteric beliefs just reviewed and receive more rational ones, since such secrets were not proclaimed on the walls of tombs nor put in writing and deposited in coffins.

CHAPTER IV - CHALDEAN SOULS

Chaldean gods, like Egyptian, were men and not "abstract personalities, who presided metaphysically over the forces of Nature". They had, too, all the faults and vices of men, though with few enough of their virtues. And yet they all seem to have begun life as suns. "Each was at first a complete sun, and reunited in himself all the virtues and faults innate in the sun", from the fructifying warmth which gives life to the raging heat which destroys it. All Chaldeans worshipped all the gods of every part of Chaldea, only some put one god above the rest and others another. But there was no divinity of established supremacy everywhere any more than in Egypt. Says Maspero: "The supreme god whom the earlier Assyriologists believed they had found, II, Ilou, Ra, no more existed than the sovereign god the Egyptologists imagined to crown the Egyptian Pantheon". Nor was there even any god of gods; one would be suzerain in one district and vassal in another. They had their trinity also, consisting of Anou, the sky; Bel, the earth, and Ea, the water; but they were not three in one, and there were two triads, one superior and one inferior. And these six were again doubled, for each had a wife, though in the council of twelve thus composed the women seem to have had little or no voice. There were special or guardian gods. "Each man was placed from his birth under the protection of a god and a goddess, of whom he was the servant, or, rather, the son", whose duty was principally to protect him from evil spirits. The Chaldeans also worshipped their dead kings.

These gods were opposed by powerful devils, not kept in Hades as in Egypt, but roaming at large like the Christian Devil, "up and down the earth", and like him and his followers were fallen angels with a like history, for they rebelled, scaled the walls of heaven, and were with difficulty flung over the parapets.

The fate of the Chaldean dead is given by M. Maspero on page 689 of his book, thus: "The dead man — or rather that which survived him, his ekimmon — inhabits the tomb, and it is to render his sojourn there endurable that they deposit in it at the time of interment or cremation (where there was cremation the ashes or charred remains were interred), the food, clothes, ornaments and arms of which he is supposed to be in need. Thus provided for by his children and heirs, he retains for them the same affection that he had when on the earth, and manifests it by all the means in his power; he watches over them, and dispels from them all evil influences. If they neglect and forget him, he revenges himself by returning to torment them in their homes. He lets loose disease upon and overwhelms them with his malediction; he is no better then than the Egyptian double, and if perchance they deprive him of sepulture, he becomes a peril not only for them, but for the whole city. The dead, incapable of gaining an honest living for themselves, are unpitying toward one another; those who arrive among them without prayers, without libations, without offerings, they do not welcome nor give alms to. The spirit of an unburied body, having neither home nor means of existence, wanders about the towns and fields, subsisting by rapine and crime. It is these who, gliding into houses at night, show themselves to the inmates under horrible aspects, filling them with terror This human survival, represented as so powerful for good or evil, was for all that only a fluid sort of being, without substance, a double analogous to the doubles of the Egyptians. With ability to go and come at will, to move itself freely through space, it could not be permanently held in the little house of brick where its body rotted; it was carried, or carried itself to the tenebrous faroff country of Arlou, situated, some said underground, others said at the eastern or southern limits of the universe". It was in this world the dead were judged and punished, by Allat, "the lady of the great country where all go after death who have breathed here below". But offenses committed against the gods, rather than those against men, occupied the attention of the court. Souls found guilty were condemned to suffer, during a life made eternal in order to enhance their misery, all manner of diseases. Those who were acquitted, however, fared little better. They were described as crying with hunger and thirst, with nothing to eat but dust and clay, shivering with cold. And if, finding this kind of life worse even than what they led in the grave, they should seek to return there, the gates were found closed upon them forever, save when quite exceptionally they were opened upon an order from the higher gods. "They retained no memory of what they did on earth. Domestic affections, memories of services rendered, all was effaced from their misty brains. Nothing floated from the wreck but an immense regret for having been exiled from this world and the poignant desire to reascend to it". But return to earth meant resuscitation, and earth spirits were on the watch to prevent that. Reincarnation seems not to have been conceived of, so far as the tiles reveal.

The Chaldean, living and dying without hope for the future, looked for happiness only during his short existence on earth. Of what was to come after it he seemed to have very dim notions, and he really seemed to care for or fear his future very little. There was among the more intelligent, it is supposed, an esoteric belief in a tolerably pleasant spiritual paradise for those who had lived good lives. But the tiles, no more than the papyrii, could be expected to tell very much of any thing beyond the exoteric and vulgar creed of the people at large. M. Maspero recapitulates what these reveal as follows: " The gods permitted no living man to penetrate with impunity their empire: whoever would mount there, no matter how brave, must make his way through the gates of death. The common man did not pretend to do that. His religion gave him the choice between a perpetual sojourn in a tomb and a seclusion in the prisons of Allat; if he sought at any time to escape from this alternative and figure to himself a different fate than either, his ideas of the other world remain vague and did not at all equal the minute precision of the Egyptians. The cares of present life absorbed him too completely to allow him time to speculate on the conditions of future one".

Writing at an earlier date than Maspero, Rawlinson affirms that the Chaldeans had no esoteric religion and cared little for the future — that after the soul, embodied in a double for the purpose, had been feasted in paradise with the good, or starved in hell with the bad, it, as pure soul, was sent up to the sun as its final home. In this he cannot be said to disagree with Maspero.

From their Chaldean kindred the Jews very naturally took many of their religious beliefs, both orthodox and heterodox. And in some way Christianity has enriched itself with the following fundamental doctrines, which are also found in the Chaldean store, namely: unintentional sin; the fall of man; the rebellion of the angels and their fall; the disastrous effect on the soul's welfare of its body not being interred according to Church usage; an unconquerable devil; an anthropomorphic god; the grave as a proper resting place for both soul and body; the greater importance of sins committed against God as compared with those committed against man, arising perhaps from the fact that God is the judge between himself and man. It is generally admitted that the Jewish religion had nothing to say of an immortal soul. And it would be reasonable to suppose that those intelligent and self-regarding Semites who descended from Chaldean Abraham discarded the poorly formulated doctrine of immortality conceived by his Chaldean fathers, because, as so formulated, it was alike repugnant to reason, taste and humanity, at once incredible and painful. But then, on the other hand, it was so very indefinite that it might very well have come in with Abraham, and then faded away of itself into what is now supposed to be nothingness, and that what little notion of it is sometimes revealed in the Old Testament is but rudimentary remains of a virtually extinct belief. However this may be, it is certain that neither Judaism nor Christianity has any reason to be proud of its Chaldean inheritance.

CHAPTER V - GREEK AND ROMAN SOULS

The Greeks and Romans, though they differed in many respects in their religious beliefs, agreed in uniting the soul and what they called its image, idol, or shade during a certain sojourn in paradise, preceded, in the case of the wicked, by more or less of preparation in purgatory; but after that inflicted a kind of second death, which severed them forever, the soul going to live in a star, or as a star, and the shade to while away its existence, such as it was, in a place of shades, which was by some thought to be in the skies above the moon and by others in the bowels of the earth. It seems to have been thought that the mere soul was incapable of enjoyment or suffering, of such at least as pertained to those half material places known as paradise and purgatory, unless in some way embodied; but, after having served these temporary purposes the shades, who, perhaps, because of the common belief in their indestructible nature, naturally arising from the fact that they were in imagination modeled on apparitions of ghosts of dead people as well as of living ones, and so could not die, were allowed to be as immortal as their nature permitted. But these, unlike what they were when figuring in paradise or purgatory, being without soul or mind, were of course not men, nor fit to people a world of any kind, quite inferior to the hardy hunting ghosts of the savage elysium, or the hard-drinking ones of the Scandinavian Valhalla, or the even more realistic spirit men of Swedenborg and modern Spiritualism.

The Greek system of belief in the time of Plato is of course best stated by Plato himself, in reading whose words now to be quoted it must be remembered that then the Universe, the heavenly bodies and the souls of men were all believed to be gods.

" Wherefore he also made the world (the God) in the form of a globe, round as from a lathe, in every direction equally distant from the centre to the extremes, the most perfect and the most like itself of all figures; for he considered that the like is infinitely fairer than the unlike. This he finished all round, and made the outside quite smooth for many reasons; in the first place, because eyes would have been of no use to him when there was nothing remaining without him, or which could be seen; and there would have been no use in ears when there was nothing to be heard; nor would there have been any use of implements by the help of which he might receive his food or get rid of what he had already digested ; for there was nothing which went from him or came to him, seeing there was nothing beside him. And he himself provided his nutriment to himself through his own decay, and all that he did or suffered was done in himself and by himself, according to art. For the creator conceived that a being which was self-sufficient would be far more excellent than one that lacked anything; and, as he had no need to take anything or defend himself against any one, he had no need of hands, and the creator did not think necessary to furnish him with them when he did not want them; nor had he any feet, nor of the whole apparatus of walking; but he assigned to him the motion appropriate to the spherical form, being that of all the seven which is the most appropriate to mind and intelligence, and so made him move in the same manner and on the same spot, going round in a circle turning within himself. All the other six motions he took away from him, and made him incapable of being affected by them. And as this circular movement required no feet, he made the universe without feet or legs".

"Such was the whole scheme of the eternal God about the god that was to be, to whom he for all these reasons gave a body, smooth, even, and in every direction equidistant from centre, entirely perfect, and formed out of perfect bodies. And in the centre he put the soul which he diffused through the whole, and also spread over all the body around about. And he also made one solitary and only heaven a circle to hold converse with itself, and needing no other friendship or acquaintances. Having these purposes in view he created the world to be a blessed god".

The reasons here given for enclosing gods in a perfect sphere apply just as well to the soul of a man after death and final riddance from both body and shade and well show the needlessness and absurdity of lodging such a soul in a body of human form, with, of course, all the needs pertaining to it.

In the Timaeus, from which the above is taken, Plato goes on to say:

"And when he had framed the Universe he distributed souls equal in number to the stars, and assigned each soul to a star; and having placed them as in a chariot he showed them the nature of the Universe". This relates to the souls before earthly birth; after death it was the same. He said that "he who had lived well during his appointed time would return to the habitation of his star, and there have a blessed and suitable existence". And a like happy fate awaited those who had lived ill, after a course of transmigrations through bodies of all kinds had purged them and made them as good as the best. And this seems to have also been the disposition of Greek souls between re-incarnations. They were sent home to the starry globes they came from. But incorrigible souls were mercifully annihilated.

Concerning re-incarnation Plato tells us in the Timaeus that belief in it was universal, and in the Phaedrus, goes into details, concerning the manner of re-birth of certain souls in this wise. "There is a law of the goddess Retribution .... the law ordains that this soul shall in the first generation pass, not into that of any other animal, but only of man; and the soul which has seen most of truth shall come to the birth as a philosopher or artist, or musician or lover; that which has seen truth in the second degree shall be a righteous king or warrior or lord; the soul which is of the third class shall be a politician or trader or economist; the fourth shall be a lover of gymnastic toils or a physician; the fifth a prophet or hierophant; to the sixth a poet or imitator will be appropriate; to the seventh the life of an artisan or husbandman; to the eighth that of a sophist or demagogue; to the ninth that of a tyrant; all of these are states of probation, in which he who lives righteously improves, and he who lives unrighteously deteriorates his lot".

Let us now turn from old to new Platonism, six hundred years intervening between the two.

CHAPTER VI - NEOPLATONISM ON THE SOUL

In the latter part of the second century there arose a school of philosophy known as Neoplatonism, which so commended itself to the instructed classes that it spread rapidly throughout the more enlightened parts of the Roman Empire, and during two centuries threatened to supersede Christianity. Its founders were as brilliant men as ever devoted themselves to such work. Its aim was to unify and at the same time spiritualize, purify and enlighten all religions without attempting to do away with any. It included a complete and perfected philosophy, psychology, theosophy and magic, as complete and perfect as great minds by long and laborious thinking and discussion could construct out of all that went before it, aided by as good inspiration and revelation as ever had come to any body of mystics, whether of Europe or Asia. But it was too fine and good for the times, and its fate goes far to prove that the wisdom of the learned should not be profaned by imparting it to the vulgar, and also that while sages and prophets may beat the bush it is always the priests who catch the bird. A school of philosophy could be no match for an organized Church, yearly growing more compact, efficient and unscrupulous, ever ready to invoke in aid of its polemics the fury of the populace or the strong arm of the government. And Neoplatonism did in fact go down before brute force. The murder of beautiful Hypatia by Bishop Cecil's mob was truly a death blow to the central school at Alexandria, and later the one at Athens was easily suppressed by a simple edict of the Emperor Justinian. By this conquest Christianity not only got rid of a dangerous enemy but also acquired that enemy's property, which she did not hesitate promptly to apply to her own use and adornment. And to-day the beautiful morality and spirituality and subtle metaphysics of conquered Neoplatonism are exhibited and vaunted as the peculiar endowment of the corporation chartered by Constantine and organized by Augustine, vouchsafed to it by God in reward for its meritorious works. Of course the acquisition lost much of its value by being combined with such dogmas as the creation of the world in time, the incarnation, and cadaverous resurrection, with their natural consequences, a combination that has proved as confusing to believers as troublesome to their teachers, who nevertheless must find it exceedingly handy to exhibit some of the choice gems of Neoplatonism, to intelligent and refined enquirers, as samples of the truth for the dealing in which the Church is sole and exclusive agent, and then when the enquirer becomes a convert deliver an inferior article of its own make. Thus Neoplatonism furnished Christianity, when sorely needing it, a brand new stock of ideas, which served it for intellectual pabulum on which to subsist in its thousand years of hibernation in the cave of the Dark Ages, and also when the spirit of criticism and doubt began to stir men's long benumbed minds, helped them take their first free steps in science and learning.

Doctrines of Neoplatonism

Ammonius Saccas, the founder of the school, left no writings, and our information concerning its teachings is derived from those of his disciples, chiefly of Plotinus, who lived in the third century A. D., which were collected by his disciple Porphery and arranged in six parts named the Enneads, of nine books each.

Revelation

The Neoplatonists were nothing if not mystics. Each for himself sought to know absolute truth by inspiration coming to him from the highest cosmic principle, while he was in a certain state of ecstasy by some supposed to be actual absorption in that principle, attainable by practices like those usual to saints and prophets. "This mystical absorption into the Deity, or the One", says Schwegler, in his History of Philosophy, "is that which gives Neoplatonism a character so peculiarly distinct from the genuine Grecian systems of philosophy".

And because of that important addition to those Grecian systems, as well as of other changes it introduced, a description of Neoplatonism properly comes in here as in orderly sequence following what has been said of Greek beliefs when Plato wrote. What those beliefs did not include three centuries before Christ they attained to by force of intellectual evolution, aided by the spread of Hindu mysticism and philosophy, three centuries after Christ, were formulated in the teachings of the Alexandrian school, and present us with the fruits of human thought in the peoples ruled over by Rome at their best and ripest stage of mental development.

The Soul

The quotations from the Enneads of Plotinus, which here follow, fully exhibit the doctrines of the Neoplatonists concerning the nature and destiny of the soul. The excuse for making them so full as they are is that except the volume of selections by Thomas Taylor no English translation of that voluminous work exists.

"And we, what are we? Are we the universal Soul, or that which approaches to it and which is engendered in time (that is to say, the body)? No (we are not bodies). Before the generation (of bodies) took place we

32

already existed on high ; we were, some of us, men, others even gods, that is to say we were pure souls, intelligences suspended in the universal essence; we formed parts of the intelligible world, parts which were not circumscribed nor separated, but which appertained wholly to the intelligible world. Even now, in fact, we are not separated from the intelligible world; but to the intelligible man there is joined in us a man who has wished to be other than himself (that is to say, the man of the senses who has wished to be independent), and finding us (for we are not outside of the universe) he has surrounded us and has added himself to the intelligible man which each of us was" (iii, 333).

"There are two faults possible to the soul. The first consists in the motive which determines her to descend here below; the second in the evil she commits when she gets here. The first fault is expiated by the very state she finds herself in here. The punishment of the second, when it is light, is to pass through other bodies more or less promptly, after judgment is pronounced against her (we say judgment to show that it is the consequence of the divine law)" (ii, 433.).

"Souls are necessarily the principle of life for all animals. It is the same with souls which are in plants. In fact, all souls issue from one principle (the universal Soul), all have their appropriate life, are essences, indivisible and incorporeal" (ii, 474.)

Relation of Individual Souls to the Universal Soul

"It must not be thought that the plurality of souls comes from the plurality of bodies. Individual souls subsist, as the universal soul does, independently of bodies, and without the unity of the universal soul absorbing the multiplicity of the individual ones, nor the multiplicity of these dividing up the unity of that. Individual souls are distinct without being separated from each other and without dividing the universal soul in a number of parts; they are united to one another without confounding themselves and without making of the universal soul a simple totality of them all : for they are not separated among themselves by limits, and they do not confound themselves with one another. They are distinct from each other as different sciences in one mind. In fine, the individual souls are not in the universal soul as bodies, that is to say, as substances really different ; they are divers acts of the universal soul . . . "all the souls from the universal soul and at the same time the universal soul exists independently of all the individual souls" (LXXX. ; of introduction to Vol. I of the Enneads, which introduction is made up of arranged fragments of the writings of disciples of Plotinus, chiefly those of Porphyry).

William J. Flagg

Descent of Soul into Body ; Reasons for it

"Thus, though the soul has a divine essence and has her origin in the intelligible world, she enters a body. Being an inferior god, she descends here below by a voluntary inclination, to the end of developing her power and to embellish that which is below her. If she flies promptly from here below she will not have to regret having taken cognizance of evil and known what is the nature of vice (without having given herself to it), nor having occasion to manifest her faculties and let her acts and works be seen. In fact, the faculties of the soul would be useless if she slumbered forever in the incorporeal essence without passing into act. The soul would not herself know what she possessed if her faculties were not, by procession, manifested, for it is action which everywhere manifests power. Without that, the soul in question would be completely hidden and obscure, or, rather, she would not truly exist, and not possess reality. It is the variety of sensible effects which makes us admire the grandeur of the intelligible principle, whose nature thus makes itself known by the beauty of its works".

"Nevertheless, they (souls descended into bodies) are not separated from their principle, from their intelligence; for their principle does not descend with them, so that if their feet touch the earth, their head lifts itself above the sky. They descended more or less low according as the bodies over which they watch have need of their cares. But Jupiter, their father, taking pity on their troubles, has made their ties mortal; he allows them certain intervals of repose, by relieving them of their bodies, to the end that they may return to inhabit the region where the universal soul always remains, without inclining towards things here below".

A Natural Law Selects the Bodies

In descending to earth each soul " enters in the body that is prepared to receive it, and which is such as it is according to the nature to which the soul has become assimilated by its disposition ; for, according as the soul has become like the nature of a man or that of a brute, does it enter a given body. What we call inevitable necessity and Divine Justice consists in the empire of Nature which makes each soul to pass in order into the corporeal image which has become the object of its affection and its ruling disposition. Also the soul becomes in her entire form the object towards which she is carried by her interior dispositions ; it is thus that she is conducted and introduced where she should go; not that she is forced to descend at such and such a moment into such and such a body, but at a fixed instant, she descends as of herself, and enters where she should. Each soul has her hour and when that hour arrives descends as if a herald called, and penetrates the body prepared to receive her, as if she were controlled and put in motion by the forces and potent attractions of which magic makes use. It is in the same manner that in an animal, nature administers all the organs, moves or engenders every thing in its time, makes the beard to grow, or the horns, and gives to the being particular inclinations and powers, when they become necessary; it is in the same manner in fine that, in the plants, she produces the flowers or the fruits at the suitable moment. The descent of souls into bodies is neither voluntary nor forced; it is not voluntary because it is not chosen nor consented to by the souls; it is not forced, since they obey merely a natural impulse, just as one is led to get married, or to the accomplishment of certain honest acts, more by instinct than by reason. At the same time there is something of fatality for each soul; this one accomplishes its destiny at this moment, and that one at that other moment. Even the intelligence that is superior to the world has also something of fatality in its existence, since it has its own destiny, which is to remain in the intelligible world and from thence radiate light. It is thus that individuals come below in virtue of the law common to all and to which all must submit. Each one in effect carries within himself that common law, a law which derives none of its force from without, but finds it in the nature of those whom it governs, because it is intimate in them. Also, all accomplish, of themselves, its commands at the appointed time, because that law impels them to do so, because deriving its force from within the very ones it commands, it presses them, stimulates and inspires them with the desire to go where they are called by their own interior vocation".

Process of Embodiment

"In descending from the intelligible world, souls come first into our sky, there they take bodies by means of which they can pass into terrestrial bodies, according as they advance more or less far (from the intelligible world). There are some who come from the skies into bodies of inferior nature; there are some who pass from one body to another. These last have not strength to remount to the intelligible world because they have forgot. Now souls differ, either by the bodies to which they are united, or by their diverse destinies, or by their kind of life, or finally by their primitive nature" (4th Ennead, 3 book).

Soul and Body — The Composite Man

"It must be then that man has for reason (for essence) something other than the soul. What prevents then that man is something composite? That is to say, a soul subsisting in a certain reason, admitting that reason to be a certain act of the soul, but that such act cannot exist without the principle

35

which produces it. Now, such is the nature of the seminal reasons. They are not without soul, for generative reasons are not inanimate; and at the same time are not soul, pure and simple. There is nothing astonishing that such essences should be reasons".

"These reasons which engender not the man (but) the animal, of which soul are they then the acts? Is it the vegetative soul? No, they are the acts of the (reasonable) soul which engenders the animal, which is a more powerful soul, and for that reason more living. The soul disposed in a given fashion, present in matter disposed in a like fashion (since the soul is such or such a thing according as she is in such or such a disposition), even without the body is that which constitutes the man. She fashions the body in her own likeness. She thus produces, as much as comports with the nature of the body, an image of the man, as a painter makes an image; she produces, I repeat, an inferior man (the man of sensations) which possesses the form of the man, his ideas, his manners, his dispositions, his faculties, but in an imperfect manner, because he is not the first man (the man of the intelligible world). He has sensations of another kind, sensations which, though they seem clear, are obscure, if compared with the superior sensations of which they are the images. The superior man (the intelligible man) is better, has a soul more divine and sensations more clear. It is he no doubt that Plato defines (in saying: the man is the soul) ; he adds in his definition : ' who makes use of a body,' because the more divine soul dominates the soul which makes use of the body, and itself uses it only in the second degree".

"I call part (of the soul) separate from the body that which makes use of the body as an instrument, and call part attached to the body that which lowers itself to the rank of the instrument".

"In effect, the thing engendered by the soul being capable of feeling, the soul attaches itself to it, giving it a more powerful life; or rather, she does not attach herself to it, but brings it near to her. She does not leave the intelligible world, but all the while remaining in contact with it, she holds suspended in herself the inferior soul (which constitutes the man of senses), she mingles herself with that reason by her reason (she unites herself to that essence by her essence). This is why that man (of senses), who of himself is obscure, is lighted by that illumination" ...

"Hence it is that the man of the last degree (the man of senses), being the image of the man who exists on high, has reasons (faculties) which are also images (of faculties) possessed by the superior man. The man who exists in the divine intelligence constitutes the man superior to all the others. He illumines the second (the man of reason), who in his turn illumines the third (the man of senses). The man of the last degree possesses in a manner the two others; he is not produced by them, he is united to them rather. The man who constitutes us has for act the man of the last degree. This one receives something from the second, and the second holds from the first his act".

"Each one of us is what he is according as the man he acts from is (is intellectual, reasonable, sensuous, according as he exercises intelligence, discursive reason, or sensibility). Each one of us possesses the three men in one sense (potentially) and does not possess them in another sense (in act) ; that is to say, does not exercise simultaneously intelligence, reason and sensibility".

"We may then say that sensations here below are obscure thoughts, and thoughts up there are clear sensations".

Why Bodies Need the Soul's Presence

"Just as a pilot steering his ship among turbulent waves, in his efforts quite forgets the danger of shipwreck, souls are drawn down (into the gulf of matter) by the attention they give to the bodies they govern; afterwards they are enchained to their destiny, as if fascinated by a magical attraction, but really retained by the powerful ties of Nature. If each body were as perfect as the universe is, it would be completely sufficient unto itself, it would not have any danger to fear, and the soul which is present in it, instead of being present there, could communicate life to it without quitting the intelligible world ".

Why Souls Descend Into Bodies.

"How comes it that the soul descends into a body, since things intelligible are separated from things sensible? — So long as the soul is an intelligence pure, impassible, so long as she enjoys a purely intellectual life like the other intelligible beings, she remains among them; for she has neither appetite nor desire. But the part which is inferior to intelligence and capable of having desire follows their impulsion, proceeds and removes itself from the intelligible world. Desiring to beautify matter on the model of ideas she has contemplated in the world of intelligence, pressed to display her fecundity and bring to light the germs that she carries in her bosom, the soul applies herself to produce and create, and, in consequence of that application, she is in some sort drawn toward sensible objects. At first she shares with the universal Soul the care of administering the entire world, without, however, entering it; afterwards, wishing to administer alone a part of it only, she separates herself from the universal Soul and passes into a body. But even then, while present in the body, the soul does not give herself entirely to it, part of her remains outside of it; thus, her intelligence remains impassible".

Punishment, Here and Hereafter

"None can escape the punishment which unjust actions merit. The Divine law (i.e. natural law) is inevitable, and has the power to carry its judgments into effect. The man destined to suffer punishment is drawn unconsciously toward it, and tossed to and fro with a ceaseless movement until at length, as if tired of striving against what he would resist, he yields himself up at the suitable place, and goes by a voluntary movement to submit to involuntary sufferings. The law prescribes the severity and duration of the punishment. Later, in consequence of the harmony which rules all in the Universe, the end of the chastisement that the soul endures comes, and with it the power to quit the place of her sufferings".

"Souls which have bodies feel by means of them the corporeal punishments inflicted on them".

"The wrongs that men commit against one another . . . they are punished for by the depravity which wicked actions introduce into their souls, and after their death are sent to an inferior place; for none can exempt himself from the order established by the law of the Universe".

"The chastisements that justly fall upon the wicked should then be attributed to that order which regulates all things as they should be. As to the misfortunes which seem to afflict the good, contrary to all justice, accidents, misery, disease, we may say that they are the consequences of former offences, for such evils are closely linked to the course of things . . . And accidents (like the falling of a house upon its inmates), which seem unjust, are not evils for those who suffer from them, if we consider how they belong to the salutary order of the Universe ; perhaps even they constitute just penalties, and are the expiation of former faults".

"Plato says that the soul's own demon conducts it to hell; also that it does not remain attached to the same soul unless this chooses (to re-incarnate) in the same condition as before. What does it do before such choice is made? Plato teaches us that the demon conducts the soul to judgment; that the latter takes after generation (re-incarnation) the same form it had before; afterwards, as if another existence then began, during the time which runs between one generation and another, the demon presides over the chastisement of the soul, and that period is less for it a period of life than a period of expiation".

"Where will the soul go when she leaves the body? — She will not go where there is nothing to receive her. She cannot enter into that which is not naturally disposed to receive her . . . Now, as there are divers places, it is necessary that the difference (of the places the soul goes to inhabit) depends on the disposition of each soul, and on the justice which reigns over all beings".

Dwelling Place between Re-incarnations of Other Souls than Sinful Ones

"What is the condition of souls which have raised themselves on high? Some are in the world of sense, the others are outside of it" (Having never incarnated.).

"Souls which are in the world of sense inhabit the sun, or a planet, or the firmament, according as they have more or less developed their reason. It must be known, in fact, that our soul contains in herself not only the intelligible world, but also a disposition conformable to the soul of the world. Now, this last being by her divers powers extended among the movable spheres and the immovable sphere, our soul must possess powers which conform to these (spheres), and each of which exercises its proper function".

"Souls which return from here below to the skies go to dwell in the star which is in harmony with their manners and with the powers which they have developed, with their god or their demon . . . When the soul returns to earth again, she has either the same or another demon, according to the life she is to lead".

CHAPTER VII - CHRISTIAN SOULS

It has often been asserted that the Persians held to bodily resurrection, and this because some of them came, in time, to depart from the orthodox custom of exposing bodies to be devoured by birds and beasts of prey (in some earlier races the survivors themselves did the eating, and from the same consideration for the purity of the four elements), so far as to bury them encased and hermetically sealed in a thick coating of wax, to protect not the body, but the earth. But the assertion is not otherwise sustained, and sentimental tenderness for the dead would sufficiently account for this practice of wax burial. The Parsees, the present representatives of the old Persian cult, do not bury in that way, but expose to the birds of prey, as of old. After their captivity among the Persians, a portion of the Jews imitated them in this wax embalmment so far as to wrap the dead in spices and deposit them in caves, where they could soon dry up and cease to offend the senses, a method inferior to the other, but superior to that of the Christians, which lets corruption work its will, trusting to some miracle to bring things into some sort of propriety and salubrity at the instant when Gabriel's trumpet shall sound the call to judgment. But the motive of these Jews was doubtless the same as prevailed with the Persians, mere sentimental tenderness, and certainly was not the preservation of Jewish corpses to take part in a Christian resurrection. And so Christianity may claim to be the first and only religion to invent and make an essential article of faith the resurrection of the corpse. The Egyptians as well as the Hindus considered the embodiment of the soul in a living human form, however fair and wholesome, for even the short season of an earth-life a deplorable imprisonment and the touching of a dead body a spiritual defilement; but the Church of Christ, which has improved on all punitive methods of ancient invention, substituting for the mild and carefully measured metempsychosis the fire-torture, and for temporary discipline with a view to reformation an eternal duration of that torture, has chained the soul a fast prisoner for eternity within a corpse, ordaining for all humanity a graveyard delivery of cadavers in every stage of decay from rottenness to dust, and for the vast majority of those cadavers (restored to completeness) eternal roasting. It is true that some of the devils of ancient times — notably that of Persia — though mortal at first, grew longer and longer lived as time wore on, and that the punishments they inflicted became more severe as wickedness increased under their régime, and it is true that whatever may have been the penal laws of any religion in its origin, a devil practically immortal and a hell practically eternal have finally encrusted themselves upon it; but Christianity from the outset made its hell eternal and its devil immortal, and if, rising up from below, as it were, belief in a spiritual body and world insists on having place in the minds of Christians and to mix and dwell with, in a most confusing way, it must be owned, the Church dogma of resurrection, that does not help the case of the dogma at all, save that by weakening faith in it it tempers its afflictive force. It belongs to Christianity and not to humanity. The other belongs to humanity and not to Christianity. They are two beliefs and not one, and if either be true the other must be false. And bodily resurrection is peculiarly the property of the Christian Church, because having its origin in an incident not known in the history of any other, nor has it been borrowed by any other, as plausible dogmas are apt to be; and if the Mohammedans hold it in an exoteric way, it was as Christians they first acquired it, for their religion in its beginning was an off-sect of Christianity, acceding to all its properties as of right. It is not forgotten here that Paul asserts distinctly that the resurrection will be of spiritual and not of natural bodies, basing his assertion on an analogy he thinks he found the planting of dead bodies to bear to the planting of living seeds. But nobody seems to have believed him, except a few who, for the very reason they did, were deemed heterodox, for the whole Christian Church went solidly for a resurrection of the very body. Here is the Christian faith as given by a Protestant preacher of high position and to be found in an American school book in common use fifty years ago:

" Scattered limbs, and all The various bones, obsequious to the call, Self moved, advance ; the neck perhaps to meet The distant head, the distant legs, the feet. Dreadful to view, see through the dusky sky Fragments of bodies in confusion fly, To distant regions journeying, there to claim Deserted members and complete the frame. The severed head and trunk shall meet once more Though realms should rise between, and oceans roar. The trumpet's sound each vagrant mote shall hear, Or fixed in earth, or high afloat in air. Obey the signal, wafted in the wind And not one sleeping atom lag behind".

But a painting by a famous artist in a cathedral somewhere in Italy does not represent the miraculous reconstruction at the last day as being near so complete. Here is a description of it:

"Then follows the general resurrection, a wonderful compartment or canto. Luca Signorelli has imagined that according to a person's good or bad deeds in this world, would be his perfection or deformity at the last day. Some, therefore, are grinning skulls, and naked cross-bones, hideously feeling about for their remaining members; others are bony skeletons lifting up their skinless eyeballs on which will never pour the day, and the yawning, hungry jaw which will now never feed upon the long offered, long rejected tree of life. The tongue, if such there be, is parched and dried up in the rootless, moistless palate, and can express fear and horror only, of all the many passions for which it once found utterance".

If we may suppose the believers who have rejected the theory of Paul and accepted the one so daintily exemplified in these two extracts, the first from the Protestant and the other from the Catholic side of the Church, to have reasoned on the question at all, several good reasons may be found in their favor and against him. An analogy is hardly an argument; an illustration is certainly none; and yet Paul's seed-planting notion amounts to less than the least of these, "Thou fool", he says, in 1st Corinthians, Chapter 15, " that which thou thyself sowest is not quickened except it die; and that which thou sowest thou sowest not the body that shall be, but a bare grain, it may chance of wheat, or of some other kind; but God giveth it a body even as it pleases him, and to each seed a body of its own", But a dead seed will never grow any kind of grain ; that part of it which sprouts is precisely what does not die, Paul may have been thinking of the notion the Pharisees had that in the teeth of a man, because they seemed to be imperishable, lay the germ of life, as a plant germ in its seed, and for which reason they withheld from cremation the bodies of children too young to have teeth that could resist fire. But there again the new life was expected to arise, not from what decayed but from what did not. Again, the learned Jew's method of raising living spiritual bodies by planting dead natural ones, leaves out of view the quick, who, at the time he wrote, since that was before the hope of a general resurrection as a daily-to-be-looked-for event had been given up, and by far the larger number of Christian converts were living people, would have played a rather important part in the scene. And if each of these had to die as he insisted that all seed must, before a spiritual body could sprout, the quick would have to be converted into dead one and all, as a preliminary proceeding. And must they not have had to be buried — planted — as well ? And then would not the delay necessary for their germination have sadly deranged the ceremonies of the great day ? But whether these considerations were found weighty or not by the foolish ones whose simple enquiries Paul was replying to, even they could tell him that it was the natural and undecayed body of Jesus that was raised from the tomb, and how in that raised-up body he declared he was not a spirit, but tangible flesh and blood, and that his resurrection was then, as it is now, the essential basis of the Christian faith, and proof of resurrection and immortality for all. Sir Stork, President of the British Royal Society, has lately told us it is the only proof. Moreover, some disposition was to be made of the dead saints who at the crucifixion left their graves and went about the streets, appearing unto many, and if Paul's theory was true such a disposition must have been rather a difficult one. If, as it requires, these saints got out of the ground they were buried in by sprouting, and came forth in his sort of spiritual bodies, they could hardly have been expected to resume their flesh, go back and lie down in their graves again, again become seed, to decay and sprout afresh when judgment day should come; and yet until then they could get no lodging in heaven or on earth, being excluded from the categories alike of the quick and dead. If they rose in their natural bodies the difficulties would have been easier got over by returning those to the graves they came from and their souls to whence they came, wherever that may have been. So Paul's argument has gone for naught, and the Christian world has today no other belief concerning the soul's immortality than as united to the very body that was buried. And notwithstanding Paul's theory of a spiritual body has place in the Church of England's burial service, the orthodox authoritative Christian belief is, and has been through the centuries that have gone by since the body of Jesus rose from the tomb, that every corpse will rise as really as it did, when at the trumpet's blast earth and sea shall give up their dead, to be reunited to their long absent souls recalled for that purpose from some place of waiting, God knows where, and thus reanimated be put on an equality with the quick who never knew the grave, in all subsequent proceedings. Accordingly the faithful who were rich enough to afford it have had themselves buried in the cloisters of churches, in the walls, below the pavements of aisles and chancels and even altars, thrusting themselves in the most unsanitary way as close under Gabriel's nose as money could carry them, and Catholics at least deem burial outside of the church-yard a deplorable calamity, damaging to the prospect of the soul's obtaining pardon for its sins, so closely is it by them thought to be connected with its shell even after death and before resurrection. As late as the year 1890 the Pope has authoritatively declared that cremation of the dead "is a detestable practice, a Pagan custom revived by evil men belonging to the Masonic sect, to obliterate the sentiment of reverence and remove the fear of death, that great fulcrum of religion".

As early as the beginning of the eighteenth century Protestants became somewhat sensitive to the ridicule, if not to the terror the dogma of the resurrection began to cause in intelligent minds, and to help the case one Thomas Boston, a learned Presbyterian divine, published in Scotland a work entitled, "The Fourfold States" in which he argued that a single particle of insensible perspiration which had escaped from a man during his life would be sufficient to serve as a nucleus for the resurrection body to form itself upon, which was going even a little further than many do, who, toiling and sweating to reconcile science with religion, at this very present time are arguing that it is only necessary, in order to have a body ready for the resurrection, that a single material germ or organized particle of the body at death should survive until then. But the latest and freshest authority on this point is to be found in a book called "The Pathway of Life" by the Rev. T. DeWitt Talmage, one of the greatest of American Protestants, on pages 24, 25, 26, of which he says:

"The forms that we laid away with our broken hearts must rise again. Father and mother — they must come out. Husband and wife — they must come out. Brother and sister — they must come out. Our darling children — they must come out. The eyes that with trembling fingers we closed must open in the lustre of resurrection morn. The arms that we folded must join in embrace of reunion. The beloved voice that was hushed must be retuned. The beloved form must come up without its infirmities, without its fatigues — it must come up".

"Oh! how long it seems for some of you, waiting — waiting for the resurrection. How long! How long! Behold the arch-angel hovering. He takes the trumpet, points it this way, puts its lips to his lips, and then blows one long, loud, terrific, thunderous, reverberating and resurrectionary blast. Look! Look! They arise! The dead! The dead! Some coming forth from the family vault; some from the city cemetery ; some from a country grave-yard. Here a spirit is joined to its body, and there another spirit is joined to another body, and millions of departed spirits are assorting their bodies and then reclothing themselves in forms now radiant for ascension".

"The earth begins to burn — the bonfire of a great victory. All ready now for the procession of reconstructed humanity! Upward and away! Christ leads, and all the Christian dead follow — battalion after battalion, nation after nation".

But a better authority with English readers would be the famous Spurgeon, who in sermon 17, second series, page 275, says:

"There is a real fire in hell, as truly as you have now a real body — a fire exactly like that which we have on earth in everything except this, that it

will not consume, though it will torture you. You have seen asbestos lying in the fire red hot, but when you take it out is unconsumed. So your body will be prepared by God in such a way that it will burn forever without being consumed ; it will lie, not, as you consider, in metaphorical fire, but in actual flame. Did our Saviour mean fictions when he said he would cast body and soul into hell ? What should there be a pit for if there were no bodies ? Why fire, why chains, if there were to be no bodies ? Can fire touch the soul ? Can pits shut in the spirits ? Can chains fetter souls ? No ! Pits and fire and chains are for bodies, and bodies shall be there. Thou wilt sleep in the dust a little while. When thou diest thy soul will be tormented alone — that will be a hell for it — but at the day of judgment thy body will join thy soul, and thou wilt have twin hells, body and soul shall be together, full of pain; thy soul sweating in its inmost pores drops of blood, and thy body from head to foot suffused with agony; conscience, judgment, all tortured; but more, thy head tormented with racking pains; thine eyes starting from their sockets with sights of blood and woe; thine ears tormented with sullen moans and hollow groans and shrieks of tortured ghosts; thine heart heating high with fever, thy pulse rattling at an enormous rate in agony, thy limbs cracking like the martyrs in the fire and yet unburned, thyself put in a vessel of hot oil, pained, yet undestroyed, all thy veins becoming a road for the hot feet of pain to travel on; every nerve a string on which the devil shall ever play his diabolical tune of Hell's Unutterable Lament; thy soul forever and ever aching, and thy body palpitating in unison with thy soul".

A catechism published in Italy, with the sanction of the Church of Rome, almost matches Spurgeon's statement, though with some variation in details.

CHAPTER VIII - RELIC WORSHIP

Kindred to corpse resurrection is a practice which is common to Buddhism and Christianity — namely, relic worship. It seems to depend on a supposed connection that binds the immortal part of a man who has died to places, persons and things which he was associated with while alive — with his habitation, garments worn and objects used by him, and especially with his grave or tomb and the body he has left in it. Whether well founded or not, the common notion that there is such a connection has been humored by the occult powers, willing to communicate with the living under guise of the dead, and the facts thus coming to its support are as numerous and common as they are indisputable. Unlike the Brahmins, to whom the touch of a corpse is a pollution calling for purifying ceremonial; unlike the old Persians, who punished severely the burying, burning, exposing to the air or casting into the water the remains of any animal, besides requiring purification after the act with such drollery of unction and drink as would, to the modern mind and stomach, at least, make matters worse — in which requirement, however, they were no droller than the Hindus; unlike the Egyptians, whose sacred writings tell us that embalming was instituted to protect from pollution the four elements; the Buddhists, and following them the Christians, have shown a saturnine fancy for things cadaverous, and made use of the most revolting object earth can show to allure God down from his throne in heaven and saints from their rest in paradise. Says Mr. Lillie, who seems to have thoroughly studied Buddhism during the nine years he gave attention to it (Buddha and Early Buddhism, by Arthur Lillie, 47): " Buddhism was plainly an elaborate apparatus to nullify the action of evil spirits by the aid of good spirits operating at their highest potency through the instrumentality of the corpse, or a portion of the corpse, of the chief aiding spirit. The Buddhist temple, the Buddhist rites, the Buddhist liturgy, all seemed based on this idea, that the whole or portions of a dead body were necessary" (Ibid., 129). Again, "Early Buddhism was an apparatus to foil the power of evil by the instrumentality of the human remains of some assisting dead saint" (Ibid., 132.)

Immaterial is it whether the Church of Rome copied the Asiatics six hundred years after the fact, or, as the Pope would say, the Asiatics copied the Church of Rome six hundred years before the fact, Christianity drew its life from the body of death as much as Buddhism did. For a long time the early Christians worked their necromancy in the Catacombs by invocations chanted over the corpses of their dead, and so much did they like it down there that when Constantine built churches above ground and provided each with the essential relics, they were loath to make use of them. Of both these great religions Lillie sums up the case thus: "Church and temple and tope have a common origin. It is not a place of worship utilized as a cemetery, but a cemetery utilized as a place of worship".

Even Protestant Luther is said to have shown a certain respect towards relics, although little of it has come down to our day as affecting any Protestant Church except that shown in the exhibition of "the elements" in the Lord's Supper, which certainly, when offered by those who believe in the "real presence", amounts out and out to necromancy, though in the others to merely a trace of it. As to the Catholic Church it is hard to detect it in any specific article of faith, but it surely cannot avoid the charge of practicing corpse-worship, when its priests even in this age of reason habitually ejaculate invocations to gods and sainted dead men over messes of bread and wine blest, exhibited and sworn to as the very body and blood of Christ, himself really present the while — really and literally so — without figure of speech, equivocation or mental reservation, attending at the call of their theurgic practice; and while in a receptacle made in the altar on which the feast is spread and actually known and called by the name of " tomb " are always kept by decree of the Church " dead men's bones and all uncleanliness". And it is only within the year of this writing that the Church has decreed that henceforth no healing done, no matter how clearly under her auspices, shall be accounted a miracle unless effected in connection with the relics of some officially recognized saint or martyr; evidently cures wrought by Christian science, mind-cure, faith-cure, spiritual mediums or mesmerizers are getting troublesomely common and quite too cheap to please Mother Church, and so, late in the day as it is, she resolves to set her mark of genuineness on but a very limited number of such cases, and leaves all others to the credit of her friend, the enemy of man, whose practice meanwhile is increasing at a rate that should make her jealous.

The Church of Rome, in her greediness for the spoils of Paganism, seems to have stolen from it more than she could well carry off, or her Pantheon well hold, and so has been forced to crowd one thing upon another in a confused way. Thus the crucifixion of Jesus is made to do duty as (1) a spectacle of torture got up to slake his Father's thirst for vengeance or satisfy his sense of justice, no matter which, the agony being all the same; (2) as a Jewish scapegoat proceeding whereby in the name of justice the just is laden with the sin of the unjust; (3) a "shedding of blood for the remission of sin", as Saint Paul puts it, a notion got from the use of blood in old magic; (4) as a meat and drink offering supposed to be pleasing to the taste of Jehovah, as such offerings were to that of all gods in early and brutal ages and is now to gods of savage peoples as well as to some tribes of those people themselves, the Fijis, for instance, with the curious variation from other sacrifices that this is offered, not by those who are to profit by it, namely. Christian sinners, but by their enemies, the Jews, who never dreamed how much good their cruel act was to do to them they hated. The feast of the Holy Communion copies the old Pagan feast of the dead, still kept in China, wherein, after the food has been merely shown to the spirits of the dead, supposed to be assisting, it is eaten up by the living. The bread exhibited on the altar recalls the "show bread" of the Jews. The wine, transmuted into blood, as blood gives a well-known potent means for helping or compelling both gods and dead men to manifest themselves. Paul seemed to think God could not be induced to remit sins, without "the shedding of blood". The priests of Baal emptied their own veins by gashing themselves with knives, in hopes it would make their god come and light the altar-fires. And in our day it is said the Kurds, by means of it, do raise some most horrid, tangible spectres. The communion ceremonies having produced on the altar the very body and blood of Jesus, his real presence is invoked and obtained by means of words said over it, just as by means of his mummy the Egyptian spirit was compelled to attend. Yet, really the only thing authorized by Jesus at his last supper with his friends on earth, was a festive commemoration of the ordinary kind. In keeping with these incongruities is the fact that the viands are spread forth on an altar that is at once a supper table and a tomb, and in its origin was a cooking range as well. So far as the celebration of mass is addressed to the Deity, it is theurgic work; so far as addressed to the saint whose dust it is chanted over or other saints, it is necromancy.

CHAPTER IX - CHINESE SOULS

Out of the belief that in spiritual form the departed still live in a spiritual world, yet still retain their interest in this, grew that system of necromantic practices which in India and Egypt, and in fact every country of antiquity, obtained acceptance among the body of the people, without regard to official religion, and which it is thought by the learned preceded all religions, as it has lived with them all, and which in a modern form bids fair to outlive one of them, at least. It is called ancestor worship, though there is little or no worship about it. In China it has attained its most notable development, and as practiced there, is most worthy of attention. Before Confucius came or Buddhism was heard of, possibly before old Taoism appeared, it existed as to-day it exists. Confucius, foe to superstition as he was, did not disturb it. Of the Kweishin, or beings corresponding to the "communicating spirits" at modern seances, he said: "We look for them but we do not see them, listen, but we do not hear them; yet they enter into all things, and there is nothing without them". " Their approaches you cannot surmise, and can you treat them with indifference ? " This teacher, who left no affirmation of belief in man's immortality, nevertheless so respected ancestor worship in the form he found in vogue, that he not only did not discourage it, but by clear implication sanctioned it, though coupling his sanction with an injunction that in its practice "no enquiry should be made concerning the nature of the spirits". Of it Professor Williams says ("The Middle Kingdom", II, 236), after alluding to the effect on the people of China of their three other so-called religions: " But the heart of the nation reposes more on the rites offered at the family shrine to the 'two living divinities' who preside in the hall of ancestors than on all the rest. Every natural feeling serves indeed to strengthen its simple cultus. In every household a shrine, a tablet, an oratory or domestic temple — according to the position of the family — contains the simple legend of the two ancestral names, written on a slip of paper or carved on a board. Incense is burned before it, daily or on the new and full moons; and in April the people everywhere gather at the family graves to sweep them and worship the departed around a festive sacrifice. Parents and children meet and bow before the tablet, and in their simple cheer contract no associations with temples or idols, monasteries or priests, processions or flags and music. It is of the family, and 'the stranger intermeddleth not with it'. As the children grow up, the worship of ancestors whom they never saw is exchanged for that of nearer ones who bore and nurtured, clothed, taught and cheered them in helpless childhood and hopeful youth, and the whole is thus rendered more personal, vivid, and endearing. There is nothing revolting or cruel about it, but everything is orderly, kind and simple, calculated to strengthen the family relationship, cement the affection between brothers and sisters, and uphold habits of filial reverence and obedience. Though the strongest motive for the worship arises out of the belief that success in worldly affairs depends on the support given to parental spirits in Hades, just as the strongest motive for worshipping God may, who will resent continued neglect by withholding their blessing, yet, in the course of ages, it has influenced Chinese character in promoting industry and cultivating habits of domestic care and thrift beyond all estimation". The gods are to be feared and their wrath deprecated, but "the illustrious ones who have completed their probation represent love, care and interest to the worshippers if they do not fail of their duties".

The author goes on to say : " The three leading results here noticed, viz., the prevention of a priestly caste, the confimation of parental authority in its own sphere, and the elevation of the woman and wife to a parity with the man and husband, do much to explain the perpetuity of Chinese institutions". After which admissions we may excuse the Professor for remarking that ancestor worship was not sanctioned by the scriptures he believed in, inasmuch as it carried filial piety too far to please Jehovah, the jealous God.

But until one knows more than this of the actual content of ancestor worship in China, he will hardly be able to understand how it should have produced the great results above attributed to it. Let us complete the account Professor Williams has given of it, and which in its shortcoming might remind one of a wheel with the hub left out.

Johnson, in his work on the religions of China, in the chapter on this Worship and in immediate connection with it, though he tells us that the whole of American spiritualism, planchette and all, have been common there in all times, is equally careful not to give us any idea of what that worship really consists in. Both writers, the one a Christian and the other a skeptic, though highly commending the worship (which by the way the Emperor once assured the Pope in an epistle was worship in no other sense than that of gratitude and respect), fall far short of telling the whole story of it, which is very much like falling short of telling the truth. But it is not unusual for men who go to foreign countries to write books about them to imitate the merchants who go to make money, and bring back only what there is a ready market for at home. At the time these gentlemen wrote American spiritualism was having a hard struggle with the two learned professions whose interests it threatened and was darkly beclouded with the contemptuous ignorance of men of science already weighted down with knowledge or conceit of knowledge beyond their power easily to carry; and it would not have been expedient to make it known that what was thus opposed and condemned here had its true counterpart on the opposite side of the world in the institution whose effects they had so much praised and which had maintained itself there with beneficent results since pre-historic days. Yet such is the truth. The Chinese worship of ancestors is, as to ceremonial, a small affair. The true content of it is nothing less than habitual and familiar communion with the dead, or what is believed to be such. A learned Chinese gentleman of the lettered class, who came to this country as attache to the Chinese Legation, gave the following account of it: The family, assembled in the ancestral hall, sit for awhile in silent meditation, exerting an earnest desire that the ancestors will communicate to them the information and guidance needed in relation to the conduct of the fortunes of the family or those of any members of it — whether a son should enter upon competitive study, whether a certain piece of property should be bought, or another sold — a certain field planted with this or that kind of grain — a certain marriage contracted or concerning any other temporal matter. Usually they have prepared themselves by twenty-four hours of fasting, or at least abstinence from fats. The simple ceremonial does not include singing or praying unless a sort of invocation written on paper and then burnt up can be called such. After the quietude and concentration of mind which is the real moving force in necromancy, theurgy, and every other branch of magic, has had the effect of inducing on the part of the "spirits "a readiness to respond, an answer is given either by planchette writing, in the way now to be described, or by trance speaking, or other modes known also to modern spiritualism, but most commonly it is by writing. A table having been covered with a thin and even layer of sand, an instrument is laid on it called a "sand pen", usually in form of a cross with a point turning downwards from the end of the longer arm and at right angles with it, for tracing the letters. At the propitious moment a boy under the age of puberty, who is present for the purpose, lifts all of the pen but its point from the table by sustaining with the back of an index finger each of the two shorter arms. This is done with the backs of the fingers as a precaution against unconscious muscular motion or conscious deceit on his part.

Here we find a true spiritual "séance" such as is now disturbing the quiet of all science, philosophy and religion, in the beneficent ancestor worship of China, whose beginning is traced back thousands of years and then lost in the dim distance of unchronicled time. As said before, it is not a religion, but merely a popular practice of one form of magic, not to save the souls, but to advance the fortunes of the members of the family, console them and promote their comfort. It had been sanctioned by both of the intruding "religions" so called, of Confucius and Buddha, and came down from antiquity in company with old Taoism. Even the Jesuit missionaries approved it, by allowing their converts to continue its practice, which is proof enough that it was a good institution and also not a religion. Little more, in fact, are either of the three other so-called religions of China really so in any sense understood by Christians.

R. H, Conwell, in his "Travels in China", quoted by Dr. Peebles in his book, "Around the World", says : "Not only do the Chinese Spiritualists believe in the same agencies and same results which distinguish Spiritualists here, but they also practice all the methods adopted in this for spiritual manifestations and a hundred others that do not seem to be known here..." "During the stay of spirits in that nether world, the lower spheres, they can rap on furniture, pull the garments of the living, make noises in the air, play on musical instruments, show their footprints in the sand, and, taking possession of human beings, talk through them".

Says Peebles himself, in his account of what he learned in China: " These Orientals have their trance mediums, mostly females; their writing mediums, using a pointed, pen-like stick, and a table sprinkled with white sand ; their personating mediums, giving excellent tests; their seers, who professedly reveal the future, and their clairvoyants; who, to express their meaning in English, 'see in the dark'. And he quotes Gonzolo, a missionary, as saying : "There is no driving out of these Chinese the cursed belief that the spirits of their ancestors are about them, availing themselves of every opportunity to give advice and counsel".

In confirmation of what had been said of the great antiquity of spiritualism in China, there is quoted a record of an Imperial decree against it by the Emperor Yao, who reigned 2337 years B.C.

This being so, and ancestor worship having kept the priest out of the house and the family out of the temple, it may be truly said that not even the great old Greeks were so little afflicted as these people have been, by temple or priest. With Buddhism to satisfy in full that craving for metaphysic which Schopenhauer doubtingly tenders as a reason for the presence of religion in the world, and ancestral worship to satisfy that more rational craving for guidance and consolation in the hard ways of that world, the vast Chinese nation has managed to get along with no religion, or next to none, very comfortably, and to live and let one another live and multiply, although having three very disputable creeds to quarrel about, in a peaceable, unchristian way, until they count four hundred and fifty millions, and this during those very centuries in which European nations were thinning themselves out by fire and sword, for the love of God and the territory of their neighbors, so effectively that in the great and fertile area of France the survivors as late as only a century or two ago, counted but ten millions. And a scanty population included within the straggling bounds of a few disjointed principalities of two thousand years ago have unified and civilized themselves and become the mightiest nation of the world, enjoying, all things considered, and as human affairs have gone since the golden age, a security, peace, order and general intelligence that is unparalleled. I say the mightiest nation, for in the resources of might China is so. General Sir Garnet Wolseley asserts that her people have all the military virtues, and could, if they would, sweep Asia clear of their annoyers and disturbers. And this American nation of ours has no adequate guarantee for the safety, of the western part of her at least, from the righteous anger of a near neighbor so endowed with latent warlike energy but the fact that that neighbor has also the virtue of loving peace. Now, this result Williams admits has been mainly obtained by the habitual practice in every family in China of what is nothing more, though somewhat less, than "American Spiritualism"; which, well considered, must bring up the question: How will so efficient a cause as this has proved itself to be on the opposite side of the globe affect the country of its latest revival and those others in which it is so rapidly spreading?

CHAPTER X - JAPANESE SOULS

Japanese civilization, they now say, is hardly fifteen centuries old, yet in that time Japanese religion, originally simple ancestor worship, underlaid, as of course, by the usual gross superstitions of earlier origin even than it, which all savages are addicted to, has been successively overlaid and the life almost crushed out of it, by Mikadoism, Buddhism and Confucianism. First Mikadoism made it a State Church in the interest of the conquering tribe that first enforced unity upon the islanders, enthroning its chief, as at once emperor of all the earth and god of all the heavens. Later came over from the Continent the finer contrived system of Buddha, and superseded in the State establishment the ancestor-cult element, and, later still, came Confucianism. Nevertheless, to the last that element has held its own in the belief of the people, and even modified the intruding faiths, or, rather, exchanged modifications with them. Each one of these imported influences has done its work in adding to and taking from the aboriginal worship, and have so deformed, disguised and covered it up, that those learned men who, in the last two centuries, have made researches into the original of it, have had tasks akin to those of the excavators in Egypt and Chaldea. At present, however, in the light of those researches, and of what is known of ancestor worship in other countries, it is not difficult to identify it with that worship, or to see that from its first absorption in Mikadoism until now it has been, despite Mikadoism, Buddhism and Confucianism, the efficient religious power working to mould the civilization of Japan, and the character of its people. That originally it was very different from the Shinto that was formed upon it, later is said to have been proved by high antiquarian authority, and yet Shinto has always carried in its bowels the original ancestor worship, and, like other systems, been sustained by it, or, rather, both have been kept alive by certain manifestations of the occult side of human nature, whose universality and persistency show them to constitute a scientific basis capable to hold up as superstructure all the religions of the world, which have never been other than interpretations, or misinterpretations of those manifestations. So in Shinto ancestor worship proper must be searched for. And for aid in doing so, here are some of the points of agreement of Japanese ancestor worship and ancestor worship in general.

(1) Gods. Aside from the Mikado, shintoism imposes on its votaries no divinities other than their own forefathers, to whom they love, as always they have loved, to address unuttered invocations, such as this: "Spirits august of our far-off ancestors, ye forefathers of the generations, and of our families and of our kindred, unto you, the founders of our homes, we this

day utter the gladness of our thanks". In pure ancestor worship all the dead are gods, and there is no god above them. And these gods are spirits and inhabit a spiritual world, while at the same time caring for dwellers in this natural one. Hirata, a commentator quoted by Hearn, says: "The spirits of the dead continue to exist in the unseen world which is everywhere about us, and they all become gods, of varying character and degrees of influence. Some reside in temples built in their honor; others hover near their tombs, and they continue to render service to their prince, parents, wives and children as when in the body. . . Every human action is the work of a god".

(2) The way of the gods. This is the literal meaning of the Japanese term Kami no Michi and of the Chinese word Shinto, the last syllable of which means way, as does Tao, the name of the old Chinese religion. The Hindus, too, have their way of the gods leading, as the Japanese one does, to a "land of the gods". In both cases it applies to ancestor worship and to the early stages of it, before, as happened in Hindustan, it was over-laid by Hinduism proper with its higher development of theism, or, as in other countries, by Buddhism. Thus the aboriginal faith is found to have given Shinto the very name it bears.

(3) The household element essential to ancestor worship shows plainly, too, in the Shinto. Hearn says: "And there is reason to believe that the early forms of Shinto public worship may have been evolved out of a yet older family worship. . . . Indeed the word ujgami, now used to signify a Shinto parish temple, and also its deity, means family God.... And to the student of Japanese life by far the most interesting aspect of Shinto is offered in this home worship". For that worship every dwelling has a room set apart called the spirit chamber, with a shelf or shrine called "the shelf of the August Spirits", on which rest tablets each of which bears the name of a departed member of the family, with the sole addition of the word "Mitama" (spirit). This chamber corresponds to the Chinese " ancestral hall".

(4) Seance, sitting. We have seen that the term Upanishad, which the Hindus apply to their very old Scriptures, means "sitting near a person". Now the name given to the Japanese medium, called in when the family desires to consult its spirits, "Nakaza" means "seat in the midst". No more than the modern Spiritualists in their circles do the worshippers, if such they can be called, ever kneel to the spirits. Their requests, which can hardly be called prayers, are preferred in a sitting posture; which again is a reminder that Pythagoras said : "You should sit when you pray". This omission of the abject devotional attitudes, common in more theistic stages of religion, is quite appropriate to a worship which has little or no ceremonial, in which the sacrifice is merely a present of food, made by children to parent, and the asking of like worldly favors in return, but especially of advice and guidance in the affairs of the family, of which all present, living or dead, are equally members. In fact in Japan, as in China,

the sitting in the ancestral chamber is very much of a family council, and very little of a devotional congregation.

(5) Concerning the modes of communication between the ancestor and his descendants, we have seen that those adopted in China are just like those we are familiar with in America. It would be safe to presume it is the same in Japan, though the authorities at hand mention only what we know here as personation, trance-speaking and tablemoving, but these are enough to identify the two quasi religions as one and the same, though the latter one is no copy of the earlier, but an original creation springing up in our Western wilds as mysteriously, and as naturally too, as in those same wilds the herb " pennyroyal " springs up wherever the primeval forest is cleared off, and pine trees replace felled oaks. But however the communications from the departed come the Japanese like the Chinese believe and obey them, and after an experience begun in pre-historic times and uninterruptedly continued until now, find them good. That they are believed, obeyed and found good of course does not prove that they come from spirits of the dead, which, however, is the firm fixed belief of the people, who avoid risk of being disenchanted in that regard by observing the admonitions of Confucius against pushing their enquiries too far. The sage who said : "Do not ask me about the next life when I cannot explain this", also said: "To give one's self to the duties due to man, and while respecting spiritual beings to keep aloof from them, may be called wisdom", and again: "Honor the gods and keep them far from you".

(6) The Phallicism found in Shinto belongs unmistakably to ancestor worship, the phallus being the most obvious symbol of paternity. It also belongs to nature worship as emblematic of fire and of the sun. But it seems that some Christian ladies, going to Japan, looked upon the emblem and were shocked, and to please them the Government in 1872 destroyed or hid away all such representations, whether floating as harbor buoys or throned in temple shrines. It is presumed the shocked ladies were Americans, for in India, where Britain rules, there has been no such interference with the worship in question, and women of the European Continent are even less disposed than those of Britain to get shocked by innocent inevitabilities. That the people peacefully submitted to the insult and degradation of the emblem of their forefather worship and of their beloved sun goddess, shows that they were very obedient subjects or had a very strong ruler; in any case, such a concession to the nerves of one people by another was unparalleled. Perhaps it would not have been made if the islanders, before making it, had tested their artillery, as they lately have done. Griffis, while rejoicing in the removal, says: " Modern taste has removed from sight what were once the common people's symbols of the god way — that is, of ancestor worship. The extent of the phallus cult and its close and even vital connection with the god way, and the general and

innocent use of the now prohibited emblems tax severely the credulity of the Occidental reader", and adds: "In none of the instances in which I have been eye-witness of the cult, of the person officiating or of the emblem, have I had any reason to doubt the sincerity of the worshipper. I have never had reason to look upon the implements or the system as anything else than the endeavor of man to solve the mystery of Being and Power".

Truth is worth some sacrifice. The veil of modesty is but a thick or thin lie, whatever may be the demerits of the thing it hides. Too much propriety has its inconveniences. There is a certain comfort in calling things by their right names, and facing bravely nature and truth. This the Japanese do, and ever have done in all the movements of life, and still manage to be a gentle, mild-mannered, pleasant and really refined people. And it would have been more creditable to the good sense of the aforesaid women to have abstained from looking at or going to see what they have been taught it was naughty to look at — in company with men — but the Japanese had not — than to have asked a forty-million nation to change its time-honored customs in respect to things sacred to them. In America, prudery is a nuisance such as it is in no other country, and sometimes amounts, when it takes the form of law, to tyranny outright. To consistently complete the work so notably begun in Japan, our good women should carry their crusade over the entire globe, and labor for the abolition of every church-spire, obelisk, pyramid and crucifix that stands; for all of these, besides being emblems of the sacred fire and sun god of Paganism, have all other phallic significance. Nor would the good work be complete until the round towers of Ireland had been razed to the earth and the columns of Stonehenge broken up to macadamize the roads. Something like a parallel to this interference with Japanese religious sentiment would be a demand upon Austria, for instance, to abolish the numerous effigies that border the roads of that country, representing in life-size and colors the death of Jesus by torture, the sight of which hurts not only the religious preconceptions of Protestant travellers, but the human feelings of all sympathetic persons who pass by, and is intended to do so.

(7) No morality. The ancestor worship that lies enveloped in Shinto had no moral law except what is written on the heart of man, and so Shinto has none. Says Griffis: " There are no codes of morals inculcated in the god way, for even its modern revivalists and exponents consider that morals are the invention of wicked people like the Chinese"; also that, "utterly scouting the idea that formulated ethics were necessary for these pure-minded people, the modern revivalists of Shinto teach that all that is 'of faith' now is to revere the gods, keep the heart pure, and follow its dictates". Lowell, writing on the same subject, says: " The gods never so much as laid down a moral code, 'Obey the Mikado' and otherwise 'follow your own heart' is the sum of their commands; as parental injunctions as could very well be

framed". And a famous expounder of Shinto, Motowori, quoted by Hearn, writes: "All the moral ideas which a man requires are implanted in his bosom by the gods, and are of the same nature with those instincts which impel him to eat when he is hungry or to drink when he is thirsty. . . . To have learned that there is no way (in the sense of moral path) to be learned and practiced is really to have learned the way of the gods". Hirata, before mentioned, says: " If you desire to practice true virtue, learn to stand in awe of the Unseen, and that will prevent you from doing wrong. Make a vow to the gods who rule over the unseen and cultivate the conscience (Magokoro) implanted in you, and then you will never wander from the way". Also, "Devotion to the memory of ancestors is the mainspring of all virtues. No one who discharges his duty to them will ever be disrespectful to the gods or to his living parents. Such a man will be faithful to his prince, loyal to his friends, and kind and gentle with his wife and children". Finally, Mr. Nose Ei, quoted by Sir Edwin Arnold, says of the followers of Shintoism : "Their ethical diction is not derived from religious writings"; and the instances he cites to show this, in Sir Edwin's opinion, "go far to prove that the Japanese really did invent an elaborate morality for themselves", based on "the eternal fitness of things" and "that revelations are not necessary to teach men to love the right and hate the wrong". But the "wicked Chinese", whom the Shintoists think may need the moral regulation which themselves do not, in the the olden time, before Confucius came to elaborate an ethical code for them, and before Buddhism had appeared to impair the original faith, held very much the same notions as these Japanese do. Lao Tsee, who lived some six hundred years before Christ, and who wrote the only authoritative statement of that faith which remains, namely, the "Tao-te-king", orthe "Book of the way and of virtue", expressed much contempt for the ethical disquisitions of his junior contemporary Confucius, and insisted on the ancient principle that "the heart of man is naturally good" and needs no moral instruction, as much as the Shintoists do, and even now the first lesson the Chinese child receives the first day he goes to school is still that maxim, "the heart of man is naturally good", to which every human heart must give an approving throb, notwithstanding Christianity has solemnly amended it by striking out "good" and inserting "evil". Probably old Robert Owen, who during thirty years educated all the children of a town of three thousand people and said he never had a bad child in his school, taught them the Chinese maxim and not the Scotch. And if Japanese children are, as travellers report, milder, gentler and better than ours, may it not in part be due to their being early imbued with this heathenish and unchristian gospel of goodness?

Older, simpler, and if you please lower than intrusive Buddhism and Confucianism though it be, there is no doubt that ancestor worship, enveloped in Shinto, has ever been the working religion of Japan, as it has been of the Hindus, Chinese and other peoples. Its value as tested by results need not be much dwelt on here, for all the world now is giving attention to them with information in aid of judgment well spread before all, which each will scan from his own point of view. A good many have come to the conclusion that, all things considered — our murdering set off against their suicides, our foeticide set off against their infanticide, and our immoral and unlawful unchastity against their lawful moral and customary departures from our standards in that respect — they are better than we, and furthermore, that in regulating sexual relations, not merely within the pale of marriage but without it, in the interest of order, health, decency and humanity, instead of disregarding those interests in futile and mischievous endeavors to suppress the irrepressible, and prosecuting nature unto outlawry, they are also wiser than we.

Ancestor worship has proved itself to be the most persistent of religions, coming earliest, staying longest, and existing in full vigor to-day; and if the Shinto is persistent it is more reasonable to attribute its persistence to the old faith that lies underneath it than to either the Mikadoism, Buddhism or Confucianism that lie atop of it. Further concerning Shintoism, Mr. Lowell, in his "Unfamiliar Japan", says:

"Buddhism, changing form or slowly decaying through the centuries, might seem doomed to pass away at last from this Japan, to which it came as an alien faith; but Shinto, unchanging and vitally unchanged, still remains all-dominant in the land of its birth, and only seems to gain power and dignity with time. Buddhism has a voluminous theology, a profound philosophy, a literature vast as the sea. Shinto has no philosophy, no code of ethics, no metaphysics; and yet, by its very immateriality, it can resist the invasion of Occidental religious thought as no other Oriental faith can. Shinto extends a welcome to Western science, but remains the irresistible opponent of Western religion; and the foreign zealots who would strive against it are astonished to find the power that foils their uttermost efforts indefinable as magnetism and invulnerable as air. Indeed the best of our scholars have never been able to tell us what Shinto is. To some it seems to be merely ancestor worship, to others ancestor worship combined with nature worship; to others again it seems to be no religion at all; to the missionary of the more ignorant class it is the worst form of heathenism. Doubtless the difficulty of explaining Shinto has been due simply to the fact that the Sinologists have sought for the source of it in books: in the Kojiki and the Nihongi, which are its histories; in the Norito, which are its prayers; in the commentaries of Motowori and Hirata, who were its greatest scholars. But the reality of Shinto lives not in books, nor in rites, nor in commandments, but in the national heart, of which it is the highest emotional religious expression, immortal and ever young. Far underlying all the surface cross of quaint superstitions and artless myths and fantastic magic there thrills a mighty spiritual force, the whole soul of a race with all its impulses and powers and intuitions. He who would know what Shinto is must learn to know that mysterious soul in which the sense of beauty and the power of art and the fire of heroism and the magnetism of loyalty and the emotion of faith, have become inherent, immanent, unconscious, instinctive".

"Trusting to know something of that Oriental soul in whose joyous love of nature and of life even the unlearned may discern a strange likeness to the soul of the old Greek race, I trust also that I may presume some day to speak of the great living power of that faith now called the Shinto, but more anciently Kami-no-michi, or the way of the gods".

Ancestor worship holds men to right conduct not merely through a fixed belief that every thought, feeling and act of the living is known to those of the dead whom when in life they most loved and revered and from whom was received the very maxims of goodness they are expected to keep, but also through an equally fixed belief that the living parents to whom at present they owe love and duty are in future to be not merely their parents, but their gods.

And here in passing, may it not be supposed that the notion common to all religions, that the powers that are on high punish sin committed here below, had its origin in this belief that the present parent is the future god, since that is just what parents are used to do. Weigh in any just balance against such an influence as this the fear of even the most modified form of the Bible hell which Christian orthodoxy permits of, or which Christian heterodoxy has of late contrived to meet the popular demand for a reasonable and credible retribution for sin, and which will kick the beam?

Shinto, says Lowell: " Signifies character in the higher Sense — courage, courtesy, honor, and, above all things, loyalty. The spirit of Shinto is the spirit of filial piety, the zest of duty, the readiness to surrender life for a principle without a thought of wherefore. It is the docility of the child; it is the sweetness of the Japanese woman".

CHAPTER XI - THE POSSIBILITY OF
A SPIRITUAL WORLD CONSIDERED

Although ghosts may well have induced a belief in a world of spirits, they go little or no ways towards proving it. They are in their nature representations and not entities, nor yet reflections, shadows, mirages of such. The supposed spirit of the modern Spiritualists is a being not only superior to, but more real and substantial than any natural man, and dwells in a habitat equally so as compared with the natural world, and the last persons to admit that its inhabitants were common ghosts would be those Spiritualists. The immortality they look for is to be enjoyed by glorified personalities in a radiant environment that is not ghostly at all. Accordingly these, when they would infer the substantial spirit from the thin and vanishing shade, resort to the supposition that the spirit disguises itself in a form, and with the costume and other accessories needed to recall to the beholder the living man of an earlier date.

How a real "revenant" (returner) from a world of spirits, if there be such, would appear no one can tell, since it must be something beyond experience or guess, but common sense says it could not appear as a ghost if it came in proper person. Some few of the opposite school, namely the materialists, whom the overwhelming evidence now within easy reach of all has convinced that apparitions do come, have put forward another supposition, which is that they are inanimate projections, reflections, shadows, mirages of living men or the bodies of dead ones. But this supposition will not bear examination. A sick man lies on his bed, or his corpse in its coffin, or, later on, in its grave, where decomposition is fast distorting it out of all likeness to anything living, while miles away an image that perfectly reproduces the same man, not in night gown or shroud, but clad, shod and coiffed as he was before he fell sick, goes noiselessly along the way. This cannot be a projection, reflection, shadow or mirage of anything whatever, for nothing like it anywhere exists above ground or below. Such appearances can only emanate from something exactly the same to the eye that is at the very time in question actually in being. There can be no shadow cast by a non-extant substance. If living or dead bodies can project images of themselves these must be simply their likenesses as they actually are. It is true that nowadays the talking ghost usually claims to be a spirit and to come from a world of spirits; but his word is worth no more than that of the shade of ancient times who proclaimed himself a god.

It cannot be doubted by any one who has read much of history that in all times men have objectively and subjectively, mentally in dreams and visions, and actually, separately and in groups and crowds, been visited by apparitions purporting to be of supernatural beings such as they were accustomed to believe in as gods. In fact, it is doubtful if any god would have remained long in popular belief after ceasing to present himself in some way to the inner or outer senses. And if a ghost proves a world of spirits, then is every god and goddess proved whose semblance ever came to earth. Priestly teachings have crowded heaven up to its zenith and earth down to its core with divinities of every degree, with angels and devils, saints and demons, while the imaginations of the people themselves have filled earth, air, fire and water, with sylphs, salamanders, undines and gnomes, all of whom have had the habit of appearing unto men. When Christianity came it found every spring in Greece in the keeping of a lesser deity, and as these insisted on showing themselves as usual notwithstanding the change in the ecclesiastical administration the new Church cunningly adopted and made saints of them, while the vulgar, being quite sure of their facts, let them be christened with new names and went on loving and believing in them as before. So the proof afforded by a spectre's resemblance to a dead person as well as that afforded by its declarations must fail because they prove too much. Another supposition which takes the ghosts to be real things and yet not spirits of the dead is put forward by some Hinduists, which is that when a dying mortal casts his body into the grave he also casts upon the air a vaporous "astral" corpse, which decays as the other does and in the same measure, and that this "shell" falling into the hands of mischievous beings of one kind or other is exhibited as the ghost. And to account for the clothing it wears the supposition is further made that the coats, vests and trousers, hats, shirts and shoes of the departed have all of them astral counterparts which are used to dress up the phantom in recognizable shape. But now let the thing thus dressed up be supposed to show itself two or three years after the death, and when the thing in the grave is looking its worst, and the astral drifting on the air looking just like it, as it must if, as said above, the two decay together, there would be presented to view something beyond measure more horrible than any ghost story tells of or mortal nerves could bear. Or if perchance one time in a thousand a corpse is shown, to indicate a death, it is a seemly one, and, serving such a purpose, can be accounted for on the theory of telegraphic representation, without need of resorting to any other. Furthermore, if the astral body decays in the same measure as the other does, must not the astral clothes rot and wear out in the same measure as their counterparts do, and if so would not the half-decayed representative of the man two or three years dead have to cover its deficiencies with astral rags ? And has such an object ever been shown, to affright the world ?

Gods and ghosts are of the same thin, spectral nature; a bullet goes through the ghost without effect, and the ancients detected a god when he walked the earth by his casting no shadow. Spectres do not tarry long. Having, in a business-like, straightforward way delivered their messages, which are usually important, as for instance, when Lord Lovatt's mounted ghost came galloping along the road to overtake a surviving friend and tell him how a paper could be found that would enable his widow to defeat an unjust claim then in suit against his estate, they quickly depart. Their interviews usually last but a few minutes, sometimes only a few seconds. Often their mission seems to be fulfilled by merely showing themselves. And in general what they communicate when they come of their own motion and not upon invocation, is of intelligible import, relates to the living and the affairs of this life, is true in statement and benevolent in intent. All which characterizes them as messengers, that is, angels, and as coming because some good overruling power sends them. Their fleeting nature of itself marks them as shows, exhibits, signals, and not active beings. Frequent failure to hold themselves together long enough to do their errands, or to speak out what they seem to have to say, or complete what they begin to tell, all go to indicate that they are produced with effort, and effort that cannot long be kept up.

Whatever may be the nature of the intelligences that lie back of such apparitions, the apparitions do not serve to reveal, but to conceal it. However real they may be as entities, we cannot know it. It is still a phantasm that is exhibited, whose nature and origin remain disguised as with mask and domino. To prove what they are they must show themselves as they are. By ghosts, only ghosts are proved. Religions and philosophies are not devised by spectres of gods or men. Such have never "gone about doing good". They are not doers in any sense. At their largest, those charged with a meaning, they are but a branch of picture language, that system of symbolic showing that was in use before words were written or spoken, that did not need to wait the coming of a Cadmus to teach it, and without being learned is universally understood.

CHAPTER XII - THE POSSIBILITY OF
A SPIRITUAL WORLD FURTHER CONSIDERED

Swedenborg's Statement.

Naturally the belief in a spiritual world has taken different forms among different peoples. So far as concerns the cosmogony and anthropology of it, that which was formulated about a hundred and fifty years ago by Emanuel Swedenborg, when he constructed his religious system known as the New Church, claiming to be guided in doing so by direct revelation made to him by Jesus in heaven, is the one which modern Spiritualists generally accept, though as respects religion Spiritualists and Swedenborgians cannot be classed together.

The work of constructing that world seems to have been neglected by the priests, and by the prophets as well, and down to Swedenborg's time left to the poets. The classic hades was a creation of Homer; the Christian heaven, hell and purgatory were imagined by Dante, and the modification of them to suit Puritan tastes by Milton; and these are by no means all who have lent their art and inspiration to that kind of construction. But no such spiritual world as that of Swedenborg seems to have been conceived by any of the poets. To put it into shape presentable to the minds of the eighteenth and nineteenth centuries an imagination like his was needed, high-soaring, wide-grasping, multifarious and untirmg, united with what those others could not pretend to, scientific and logical acumen. In a remnant of one lifetime he completed a system which all who have the energy to read it in its voluminous details must wonder at. Through more than sixty volumes (printed and unprinted) he labored to buttress its weak points and gloss it with plausibility; and if the theory of a spiritual world such as he has left cannot bear examination none can. No suspicion of imposture, or monomania, can arise in the mind of one who fairly reads his writings. As a wise, honest and sane man it was that he claimed to have talked face to face under the very dome of heaven with the Lord and Ruler of the whole universe even to its remotest star, who was none other than our own Jesus of Nazareth ; and he had as much right to do so as Moses had to say he talked with Jehovah in the burning bush, or Mahomet that Gabriel came to him in the cave. Nor were signs and wonders wanting to attest the authenticity of his commission, such as his father, the good Bishop Swedborg, by authority of the whole Christian Church, Catholic and Lutheran, had taught him "imported verity". Though he was far from obtrusive of his miraculous gifts, and relied largely on logic and the authority of the Bible to prove his teachings, usually in fact supplementing his revelations with them.

The spiritual world of Swedenborg was as natural as our own, in every proper sense, though he distinguished them from each other as natural and spiritual. It was in time and space, and perceivable by senses; therefore phenomenal, not transcendent. He tells us that all go immediately after dying into the "world of spirits", a department of the spiritual world, where "some remain for only several weeks"; " some for several years, but not more than thirty" (Heaven and Hell, S. 426), and that "things have succession and progression in heaven as in this world", though instead of ideas of time such as we have the angels have only ideas of state. "To them all is state and change of state". And it is the same as to ideas of space. The calling it state does not prevent it from being space as we conceive it, however, for after saying that into his heaven come all those fit for it who have lived on any of the myriads of earths that fill the universe, all of whom are peopled as our own is, he adds, as if the question arose in his mind: how all these could be lodged. " It has been given me to see the extent of the heaven which is inhabited and also of what is not inhabited; and I saw the extent of heaven not inhabited was so great that it could not be filled to eternity, even if many myriads of earths were given and as great a multitude of men in each as there are in ours" (Ibid, S. 419).

Another question which will occur to the reader seems not to have occurred to him, which is: can any part of space, or the whole of it even, remain unfilled for eternity when an infinite universe is during all that eternity breeding emigrants for it and pouring them in? Again, he says of heaven : "Although in heaven there are spaces as in the world, still nothing is there according to spaces, but according to states" (Heaven and Hell, S. 198.) Hell also is a place.

We are informed that " in a word the whole heaven and the whole world of spirits are as it were excavated beneath, and under them is a continual hell" (Ibid., S. 588.). This would seem to make hell no larger than heaven, though it should be vastly more so, since he tells us no one ever comes out of it, and then plainly implies that those who go in there greatly outnumber those who enter heaven, by this text, which in that connection he quotes: " Wide is the gate and broad is the way that leads to destruction and many they be who walk through it, narrow the way and straight is the gate which leads to life and few there be who find it", following it by this of his own : "That the way is narrow which leads to life is not because it is difficult, but because there are few who find it" (Ibid., 534). But the case is somewhat helped by letting into heaven all who are lucky enough to die in infancy (blessed be measles, mumps and whooping-cough therefore !), otherwise the disproportion between the populations of the two places would be greater. And the inhabitants of the spiritual world, whether angels, spirits or devils, have senses just like ours. On this point he says: "From these things it may be evident that the spirit of man is equally in a form, and that it is in the human form, and that it enjoys sensories and senses as well when it is separated from the body as when it was in the body, and that all of the life of the eye, and all of the life of the ear, in a word, all of the life of sense which a man has, is not of his body, but of his spirit in them, and in their minutest particulars. Hence it is that spirits as well as men see, hear, and feel, but after being loosed from the body, not in the natural world, but in the spiritual ; the natural sensation which the spirit had when it was in the body, was by the material which was added to it; but still it then had spiritual sensation at the same time, by thinking and willing" (Ibid., S. 434.).

Swedenborg's learned disciple, the Rev. Chauncey Giles, goes even more into details in setting forth the sensuous nature of the spirit. He says, in an address delivered in 1890 before the convention of the "New Church" at which he presided:

"The New Church regards the spirit in an entirely new way. According to its doctrines the spirit is the man himself in human form, and the seat of all his power and life. It is organized of spiritual substances, as the material body is organized of material substances, and possesses all the organs, external and internal, in general and particular, that compose the material body. It has a head, trunk and limbs, it has eyes and ears, a brain, and face and vocal organs, heart and lungs, arteries and veins and nerves. Every organ performs the same relative function that the material organs perform. The spiritual lungs breathe a spiritual atmosphere; the heart propels a spiritual blood through arteries and veins; the nerves give sensation and power; the hands grasp spiritual objects and the feet walk upon a spiritual earth. The eye opens to the light which flows from the spiritual sun, and the ear vibrates in harmony with modulations of the spiritual atmosphere. As a whole and in each least part the spirit is in the human form. The common idea had been that the body was first formed and then the spirit was breathed into it, as men make an engine and set it in motion by steam. The new doctrine teaches that the spirit itself molds the body into its form, weaves its fine and delicate texture in its own loom and clothes itself in every least part with it, making it a medium of communication with the material world, the home in which it dwells, a complicated and miraculous instrument, adjusted with infinite precision to all the forms and forces of matter, to gain natural ideas and delights to serve as material for the development of the affections and the intellectual faculties. But it is merely a temporary service. The material body renders the same service to the spirit that the husk does to the corn, the chaff to the grain".

Such a spiritual man, a very duplicate as he is of the natural man of the natural world, must needs have a spiritual world to live in that is a very duplicate of that natural world. Given the man, the world must follow. But our prophet has not left this to logical inferences ; he tells us expressly that it is so, thus:

"What those things are which appear to the angels in the heavens cannot be described in a few words; for the most part they are like the things on the earth, but more perfect as to form, and of greater abundance " (Heaven and Hell, S. 171.). Only they are not similar in essence, as those are from the sun of heaven and these from that of this world. "When it has been given me to be in company with angels, the things which are there have been seen by me altogether as those which are in the world; and so perceptibly, that I knew no otherwise than that I was in the world, and there in the palace of a King" (Ibid., S. 174.). Again, "In the spiritual world, or in the world where spirits and angels are, similar things appear as in the natural world, or where men are ; so similar that as to the external aspect there is no difference. There appear there plains, and there appear mountains, hills and rocks, and between them valleys; moreover also waters and many other things which are seen on earth. . . . Such being the similarity between the spiritual world and the natural world, therefore man after death scarcely knows otherwise than that he is in the world where he was born, and from which he has departed; for which reason also death is called only a translation from one world to another like it" (Ibid. S. 582.).

Concerning garments, habitations, etc., we have: "Because angels are men and live with one another as the men of the earth do, therefore they have garments, habitations, and other like things, yet with the difference that they have all things more perfect, because in a more perfect state" (Ibid., S. 177). "That the garments of the angels do not merely appear as garments, but that they really are garments, is evident from this, that they not only see them, but also feel them; and also that they have more garments than one, and that they put them off and put them on, and those which are not in use they preserve; and when in use they reassume them; that they are clothed in various garments has been seen by me a thousand times" (Ibid., S. 181.). These garments, it seems, are gifts of the Lord, who also gives to the devils in the hells to be clothed, lest they should appear naked, though these can only wear what is ragged, squalid and filthy.

As to habitations, he further says: "As I have often spoken with angels, face to face, so often I have been with them in their habitations. Their habitations are altogether like the habitations on earth, which are called houses, but more beautiful ; in them are parlors, rooms and bedchambers in great numbers ; there are also courts, and round about are gardens, shrubberies and fields. Where they are consociated the habitations are contiguous, one near another, disposed in the form of a city, with streets, ways and public squares, altogether in likeness of cities of our earth" (Ibid., S. 184.). We also learn that all the necessaries of life are given gratuitously to the angels; "they are housed gratuitously, they are clothed gratuitously, and they are fed gratuitously" (Ibid., S. 393.).

All the angels and all the devils, thus all the inhabitants of the spiritual world, are men who have lived and died on the various earths of the universe. Swedenborg was instructed to say: "That in the universal heaven there is not any one angel who was so created from the beginning, nor in hell any devil who was created an angel of light and cast down; but that all, both in heaven and in hell, are from the human race; in heaven those who lived in the world in heavenly love and faith, in hell those who lived in infernal love and faith" (Ibid., S. 89.). He elsewhere calls the earths "the seminaries (breeding places) of the spiritual world" (Ibid., S. 583.).

What portion of space is occupied by the vast spiritual world, with its heaven, hell and world of spirits, and into which those breeding places of angels and devils will while they last continue to pour inhabitants, we are not told, but learn that in the more elevated places of the spiritual world are the heavens, in the low places there is the world of spirits, and beneath the latter and the former are the hells, also that " heaven in the whole complex resembles one man" (Ibid., S. 59.). Though "the angles indeed do not see heaven in the whole complex in such a form, for the whole heaven does not fall into view of any angels" (Ibid., S. 62.). "There are three heavens, and those most distinct from each other; the inmost or third, the middle or second, and the ultimate or first. They follow in succession and subsist together as the highest of man, which is the head, his middle, which is his body, and the ultimate, which is the feet" (Ibid., S, 29.). Which two last passages, and many more that might be quoted, show that Swedenborg's discovery was not of a globular world like the spheres of our visible heavens, but one in the human form, really and not figuratively so. This must be kept in view while the possibility of such a world is considered. For the same purpose we should remember that according to our seer " the natural world exists and subsists from the spiritual world, altogether as an effect from its efficient cause" (Ibid., S. 88.). Which is also the theory of Professors Balfour Stewart and Taite in their book, " The Unseen Universe". And the most plausible one it is if we assume that the one world is a duplicate, in a different substance (by which term we are to understand "material", or "stuff"), of the other, which is also assumed in every other formulated belief in a spiritual world, by whomsoever held.

But, quite aside from any of these, it seems clear that any plausible theory of a spiritual world must assume that one who passes out of this earth life to become a citizen there arises from his cast-off material body a complete man, complete in all parts of him, having head, trunk, limbs, brain, heart, lungs, liver, and all other viscera, organs and members, the assemblage of which and their combined activities, with the resulting desires, passions, thoughts and volitions, make the man. It seems clear, too, that to fit such an inhabitant, as a habitat and environment possible for him to dwell in, the spiritual world must be in all essential respects a duplicate of the one he was born into and lived and died in. Such considerations seem to have been held in mind by all constructors of such worlds, and not forgotten even by the poets. The Scandinavian ghost, drinking ale out of his enemy's skull, must have a complete set of organs, or no joy could come to him from the glutting of his vengeance or the quenching of his thirst, and the spirit of the Red Indian of America must have the same in order to chase, kill and eat his game, as well as to digest it.

As said before, the enlightened pagans of antiquity also recognized the necessity of giving the soul some sort of a body to feel in, and hence the shade of which we read so much, and which had no other use.

CHAPTER XIII - THE POSSIBILITY OF A SPIRITUAL WORLD FURTHER CONSIDERED

The considerable space given in this chapter and the two following ones to Swedenborgianism and Modern Spiritualism should be excused on the ground that as already suggested they stand for all forms of ancestor worship, the fundamental religion of all mankind, and that in examining them we are inspecting the foundation of all religion. This chapter, however, and the next may be skipped by the impatient reader without serious breach of the book's chain of argument; but if he do so he will be apt to return to them later. Notwithstanding Swedenborg's insistence on the close likeness of his Spiritual World to our natural one, the differences between them are enormous. Ours is but eight thousand miles in diameter, his is large enough to hold all the dead of the whole universe, that have ever lived and died, or that ever will. Ours is a globe, his is in form a man. Ours revolves round a sun and has nights and days, moves on a tilted axis and has its seasons, his has a fixed sun that is always in the east. Ours has a soil, rather an important part of it, since to till that soil, so we may live and not starve to death, keeps us laboriously busy; his may have one, but there is no account of its being tilled. Ours is a place of temptation and transgression, his is a court of justice and a prison in part, and in part a paradise of office-holding angels, who he assures us are wonderfully happy, without telling just how they are so. The state and fate of all adults who go to his are made up here below and can never be changed ; the good become angels forever and the bad devils forever. All is very simple; no appeal, no pardon, no change.

Up there we are told the angels are kept busy enough, but it is not in productive avocations. Concerning what their employments are we are told that they are "innumerable " but mostly administrative, "for there are ecclesiastical affairs, there are civil affairs and there are domestic affairs" (Ibid., 388.) ". There are societies whose employments are to take care of infants; there are other societies whose employments are to instruct and educate them as they grow up; there are others who in like manner educate and instruct boys and girls" (Ibid., S. 391.). "There are others who teach the simple good " and "the various Gentile nations". There are others who defend novitiate spirits " from infestations by evil spirits". "There are some also who are present to those who are in the lower earth; and also some who are present to those who are in the hells, and restrain them from tormenting each other beyond the prescribed limits; there are also some who are present to those who are raised from the dead".

Thus the outcome of this universe is a world where the larger part of its population after judicial trial and also " exploration " of the interiors and a judgment based partly on a certain state of the affections and partly on overt acts resulting from it, are imprisoned for eternal life in prisons subterraneously excavated under beautiful and sublime mountains whereon the angels who have been their triers and moral vivisectors and after that their turnkeys as well, dwell in heavenly joy, which the nearness of the damned seems no more to disturb than did the groans of prisoners chained in dungeons beneath castles in olden times disturb the serenity of my lord and his retainers who feasted in the halls above. Classified rudely the occupations of these angels are those of civil and ecclesiastical rulers and administrators, jailors, dry-nurses, teachers of theology to the various Gentile nations, exorcisers of "evil spirits", guardians of mortals in the flesh, and ushers of newly arriving spirits. For the performance of all these duties except those of the civil and ecclesiastical administrations as many angels as would equal in number the product by the earths of the universe during a single generation of time would surely suffice, because the subjects of their care do not exceed n number, we are told, the incomers during not more than thirty years — in which time those needing it will have completed their growth and education and found their way to heaven or hell — while as to those in earth life needing guardianship they would not average in length of years more than about the same time. And the foregoing duties being provided for, the remainder of the enormous population of angels accumulated during infinite ages in the past have for their only occupation the administrative duties of Church and State in the heavens, and the keeping order in the hells. The Church services (where the angels are the worshippers) need not employ more than one in a thousand, and as to the number required down below, it is to be presumed that the details for the disagreeable duty of keeping ragged and ill-smelling prisoners in order must be as small as possible and their watches as short, especially since to help them in their duties, they are allowed the aid of a corps of devils selected for their superior cruelty. "Wherefore the more malignant are set over them as governors, whom they obey from fear" (Heaven and Hell, S. 220.). So that the occupations of the innumerable hosts of angels accumulated during eternity, all the worlds in the universe contributing to their production as "seminaries", consist in caring for the human product of those worlds yielded during a scant generation of time, and in ruling over one another as civil and ecclesiastical officials during time without end. Why they need so much ruling is not revealed, nor how they manage to be, as is revealed, both very busy and very happy. Thus much for the constitution of the supposed Spiritual World, now for its content. The world discovered by

Swedenborg is essentially a religious one; but his fall of man, original sin, trinity, atonement, faith, justice, mercy, salvation, free-will and their final outcomes, heaven, purgatory and hell, differ from those of all other creeds. In S. 424 of "Heaven and Hell " we learn that "man is born into every evil as to the will " ; that he is nevertheless capable of being reformed by instruction if only his evilly-born will will so will, which instruction is based on a hidden sense in the Jewish and Christian scriptures that was by their authors so long and so well hidden that it was not found out until he came to discover at once it and the world it relates to. But no amount of instruction can alter a man's destiny unless he gets it in earthly life, or dies an infant or excusable pagan, etc. The angels have a way of searching his interiors and so finding out just the state of his affections, whether he loves God and his neighbor or himself; if himself he goes to hell forever. And this even if he loves also "his own", who, specially, are his children and his grandchildren, but generally all who make one with him, whom he calls his; for to love these is the same as to love himself. Amongst those whom he calls his own are likewise all who commend, honor and pay their court to him. To the unilluminated it would seem that a man who loved his family, friends and dependents, would make a good citizen enough for all practical purposes, since from the interlacing of families and other civic relations, all the world must thus get loved, if not by everybody yet by somebody, so there would be in a world of such loving friends enough to do for all every needed office of kindness and supply every needed thmg, yet it is not so; one with a love thus limited goes to hell without remedy. The examination of the interiors is done early after the spirit's arrival in the vast intermediate state and place called " the world of spirits", where are also carried on certain judicial enquiries concerning the man s overt evil acts, which last seems hardly necessary though, since the investigation of the interiors of him have already settled his destiny. These proceedings are by no means summary either. Of one branch of testimony we read, "the manifestations continued sometimes for hours together". Memorandum books were " opened and read before them (the culprits), page by page". Again, "and what was wonderful the letters and papers which passed between them were read in my hearing, and it was said that not a word was wanting". " In a word, all evils, villainies, robberies, artifices, deceits, are manifested to every evil spirit, and brought forth from their memory, and they are convicted; nor is there any room for denial". Considering the time and trouble which these long criminal trials must require, and also that to judge the souls of a whole universe billions of causes must be disposed of daily, it must be admitted that some of the angels at least are able to keep busy. Quite in accordance with the selfacting, self-sustaining, co-operative system of criminal discipline that prevails in the spiritual world, the condemned spirits, now become perfect devils, "cast themselves down into hell", and when they get there go to tormenting one another, each performing the double part of devil and sinner. Perhaps they go thus willingly because they have learned, what the reader soon will, that Swedenborg's hell is not wholly without its compensations, nor his heaven quite without its drawbacks. Here are some of the compensations:

First. There is little or no law in hell. It is only when its people torment each other beyond a certain reasonable measure that a squad of angels goes down, and with the help of some of the "more malignant among them", called in as a sort of special constables, re-establishes order.

Secondly. Though to the angels the stench of the hells seems vile, yet we are told that to the devils themselves it is not at all so; and by analogy we may infer that the rags they wear are to them comfortable and decent clothing.

Thirdly. The devils are allowed the companionship of their families and friends and all the comfort they can find in stealing one another's wives — or having their own stolen — adultery being their chief delight and occupation.

Finally, he reports that the devils themselves, who are really the only parties concerned, feel happy where they are and would not go elsewhere if they could.

Certainly, considering the times he lived in our seer deserves credit for the consolations he allows his devils, while as to his angels — yes, as to his angels — let him who thinks he can devise a mode of future existence for disembodied men that shall bear in its detail even slight criticism from the point of view of common sense, take up the pen and write. Like all who have heretofore attempted it, he will find his heaven more difficult to contrive than his hell; possibly because man-made worlds, celestial or infernal, from the very limitations of man's nature must always be modeled on this, and in this we know a good deal about torment and a very little about joy. The task of him who would imagine and in detail describe an universe could hardly be less than that of creating one, and it is therefore quite beyond the powers of man or spirit. Here is a specimen of the difficulties of it:

Swedenborg having endowed the people of hell with the ability to indulge in sinful love was bound in logic to give the people of heaven the analogous ability to indulge in sinless love; and this he does in his "Conjugial Love", as well as in his "Heaven and Hell", which last, in order to distinctly show what he meant, I quote (S. 402) : " Conjugial delight, which is a purer and more exquisite delight of touch is more excellent than all those (other delights of sense) on account of its use, which is the procreation of the human race, and thence of angels of heaven". Having gone thus far a mighty problem arose, to wit, how to deal with the product of heavenly, letting alone hellish, love-making, which he solved to his own satisfaction at least, by making his angels, though loving, sterile, except that they are able to beget and bear what he calls "goods and truths", from which it maybe inferred that his incontinent devils are only prolific of what he calls "evils and falses"; which, however, still leaves for solution the question, what kind of things those goods and truths, evils and falses are that come of human begetting?

Further to show that Swedenborg's theology in its articles of faith is different from every other; he has no original sin, but instead an original sinfulness, from which the victim of it can be saved only through receiving and profiting by a course of instruction in the Bible's arcane meaning as above mentioned. And he allows no justification by faith, but only a reformation by means of such instruction which must be effected during earthlife or never at all. Man goes to heaven or hell, not because they are places of punishment or reward, but because fate ordains it so, perhaps, or as a theological necessity. Punishment just attaches itself to sin as it does in the Hindu system, and will not be shook off, by force of a law which, like the law of "Karma", is very labor-saving, if not so discriminating or so mild as that.

There is no theological justice to be vindicated, either by the vicarious sufferings of Jesus or the eternal burning of such as can not or will not believe the story of them.

Nor is there any divine wrath to be appeased by anybody's suffering. Neither mercy, justice nor wrath play any part in this prophet's revelations, nor in the Bible as he has interpreted it.

As in all other systems, the Almighty does the best he can.

Religious services are continually held in heaven.

There is no resurrection of the body, nor any such last day judgment as Christians of other sects believe in.

As there are no angels in heaven who were not once men, like ourselves, so except a rather imperfect trinity, there is no hierarchy of celestial birth, no archangels.

Neither Lucifer nor Beelzebub, nor Satan nor other pagan god does duty as the one omnipotent devil in Swedenborg's hell, any more than in Mohammed's.

Finally, he does not withdraw his theology from the criticism of reason, but rather invites it. His authority for it is that it was revealed to him by Jesus of Nazareth, now the Ruler of the Universe, in thousands of interviews had with him in heaven, which, though as good authority as any creed can claim, has obtained as yet but small acceptance, but his report of things seen and heard by him in the spiritual world, its manners and customs, soil and climate, occupations and productions, and the nature and constitution of the spiritual man, has gained great acceptance in their character as formulations of the old vaguely but universally held belief now being considered. They make up the best working hypothesis by far yet put forward for investigators of modern spiritual manifestations, which is a precious boon to all the millions who are classed as such, and is not without value to other searchers into occult nature now working hard to find out a better.

In "The True Christian Religion" (S. 829), where the condition of the Mohammedans in the spiritual world is described, we find the following: "And because Mahomet is always in their minds in connection with religion, therefore, some Mahomet is always placed in their view; and that they may turn their faces towards the East, over which the Lord is, therefore he is placed beneath the middle, occupied by Christians. It is not Mahomet himself, who wrote the Koran, but another, who fills his place; nor is it always the same, but he is changed. Once it was one from Saxony, who, being taken by the Algerians, became a Mahometan. He, because he had also been a Christian, was led several times to speak with them of the Lord, that he was not the son of Joseph, but the Son of God himself. That Mahomet was afterwards succeeded by others. In the place where that representative Mahomet has his seat there appears a fire, as of a little torch, that he may be known ; but that fire is conspicuous only to Mahometans. " Elsewhere we are told that this "representative Mahomet" was set up to prevent the disorders that would otherwise arise among Mahometan spirits on their first arrival, and who, as they came trooping in by tens of thousands, clamored to be shown their beloved prophet, not knowing he was long ago deposed from his seat for misbehavior.

It seems there was like trouble with the Jews, who came clamoring for "father Abraham", and that to cheat them also in the interest of order and quiet a "representative Abraham" was set up and shown to them, the original being, as it happened, like Mohammed, undergoing discipline and deprived of his place.

These two examples of systematic deception on a vast scale do not seem at all to have shocked the moral sense of the narrator of them, nor at all to have shaken his faith in the veracity of the angels in other respects. So that when he was presented to one who told him he was Jesus Christ, Lord and Ruler of the Universe, he did not suspect he was being fooled as he had seen the Mohammedans and Jews fooled, nor that some unimportant spirit was dramatizing before him as a representative Christ, nor that the voluminous disclosures that representative made to him, as well by word of mouth and face to face as by angelic commissioners sent to show him round, concerning the newly discovered doctrines of the New Church and, more than that, the very arcana of Nature, might be mere fables. The which resolves his long, far and frequent journeyings through the world of spirits into phantasmagoria of the subjective kind.

Swedenborg's revelations have great value to the student of such things, as being modern and within reach of investigation. The visions that came to him, and the sights he went to spiritual lands to see, date only a century and a half back, and were promulgated in broad intellectual daylight. Nothing was done in a corner. As a learned, scientific and practical man he was well known to all such throughout Europe. His good and pure character, his abilities and acquirements are testified to in the writings of his contemporaries in a way that leaves no room for doubt that he was as fit to receive truth from supernatural sources, if there be such, and to reveal it to the world as Zoroaster, Mohammed, Pythagoras, or any other mortal who ever dreamed or wrote. He can be got at, seized, handled, weighed, measured and tested better, perhaps, than if he lived now, for a certain interval of time is required for a good view of any historic character. He bears examination well, though his religion does not, and while the one is not doubted the other is to the world at large but rubbish. Or if now and then a reader, struck by the marvellous vigor of his writings, goes far enough into them to get at their meaning, he must stumble over, as he goes, absurdities like those of which some few are pointed out in this and a former chapter that finally make him lay them by, not without wonder and perplexity that a man who could so write should have written so. And at the same time that his teaching is thus contemned, hundreds of millions of both the ignorant and wise either actually believe in some form of it, the religion that was set up by St. Paul, or think they do, or else are just now and but slowly finding out that they do not. Yet the subject of Paul's visions and teachings lived so long ago and so obscurely that learned men doubt if he ever lived at all ; while the record of his sayings and acts is known to have been in the hands and keeping of forgers by vocation since the time when, by the votes of a very inferior body of men, it was made legal tender as the Word of God.

So far as we have any good account of their beginnings, all religions and all their great embranchments and engraftments have had a like origin, however different their contents. None has been by the god of it given directly to mankind, but each has come through an intermediary prophet, having natural or acquired receptivity for so-called supernatural inflow, and also miraculous powers, so called, to exhibit as sanction for his authority to speak for God and control man. Such were Zoroaster, Pythagoras, Moses, Saul of Tarsus, Mohammed, Boehme, and such was Swedenborg. No devotee of any faith can trace the sources of it further back than to some such intermediary, nor can this last trace further back than to something lying within his own self the revelation he transmits, be it given to him by intellectual illumination, symbolic visions or talking ones, clairaudience, clairvoyance, automatic or direct writing, trancespeaking, or whatever other of the now wellknown and well known to have been always common methods by which the hidden world speaks to the manifest one the medium was adapted to. The mystic, already religious, threading the path of contemplation, in search of the source of his being, already believed to be a god, in hope to attain to union with it, comes upon his own very self (but his inward self) as objectified by itself in form of that god or his messenger, and forthwith bows down before and worships himself; and then whatever revelation is thus vouchsafed to him he communicates to the world with the zeal that comes with absolute conviction, as the absolute truth all men long for, to meet with more or less acceptance according as time, place and circumstance may suit. In a smaller way lesser prophets have had their visions, illuminations, etc., in countless number as auxiliary revelations, enuring to the benefit of their preconceived ideas, and either really or by force of construction redounding to the glory of their Church.

Real prophets have so abounded that there is no need to suppose false ones, and in judging a given revelation the idea of imposture may generally be put aside, as certainly it may be — nay, must be — in Swedenborg's case. None but a member of the little "Church of the New Jerusalem " will believe that its founder went to heaven, and there, person to person, got his instructions from the Lord of the Universe, though many enough will, in the light of our present knowledge, be willing to admit that he thought he did, being made so to think, however, by subjective causes working wholly within him. And imposture not being a necessary supposition, yet error, inconsistency and absurdity being apparent, the inference must be that fallible man is at the bottom of the whole business, and not infallible God.

Swedenborgianism, coming in the regular way by which all religions have come, and having a content certainly more rational and credible than any, being nevertheless condemned by the age to which it is submitted for judgment, all others must be condemned, and if any newly contrived one is to obtain favor it must arise in a very different way and be a very different thing. A revelation concerning a future state or world, to be worthy of belief, or even of attention, should be as full, precise and detailed as accounts from a continent across the ocean are expected to be. And if we are to guide our steps in this world by light coming from another, that light should shed as clear a ray as the one we already have here. Swedenborg seems to have appreciated all this, for he worked hard and voluminously at the details of his plan as if in hopes to make it hold itself together, but with an opposite result, for the more details of it are given the easier it is to criticise, and while the established faiths it was expected to overturn find a measure of safety by hiding their heads in the clouds of obscurity and indefiniteness this newly proposed one has its weakness in being too clearly explained and defined. Swedenborg came too late and did his work too thoroughly for it to prevail either against old beliefs, held to because they are old and therefore deep-rooted in the mental and sentimental habitudes of believers, or against the unbelief of free-minded men.

CHAPTER XIV - THE POSSIBILITY OF A SPIRITUAL WORLD FURTHER CONSIDERED

The spiritual World of Modern Spiritualism.

Concerning what becomes of the souls of men after death the different religions have each a different story to tell, or if, perchance, any two can by construction be made to agree on this point they must differ on others, else they would be not two, but one. Now, Divine revelations cannot be allowed to differ on any point; that is a privilege accorded only to human ones. It is essential to a communication coming from an Omniscient deity that it tell the truth, the whole truth, and nothing but the truth, and, therefore, of all the many " other worlds " that have been revealed to dwellers in this, only one at most can be the real one. But as the sacerdotal keepers of the archives of each tell their devotees that their own is that very one, no inconvenience results, and each sect of believers is complacent in the steadfast faith that all the world is lied to but themselves. But he who rummages the records concerning these revelations until he finds out, as he will if he rummages deep, that all are from one and the same occult, and, to the vulgar, miraculous source, in short, that all come in the same way and are proved in the same way, will criticise them all as if coming from one witness, and to him it will be the same as if a single person claiming to know all about a given matter in dispute should tell as many different stories about it as are revealed religions in the world, and be forced by his reason to deny, not merely all save one, but all without exception, also to deny that any revelation coming from such a source is competent to prove anything whatever, least of all, fitly serve as a rule of human conduct, for the first principles of evidence teach that a witness who tells two different stories about the same thing is not to be believed as to either of them, nor as to anything else, and, even more, teach that a witness found to be false in merely one detail of his statement must be deemed false in all. Accounts of the spiritual world of our modern Spiritualists such as are generally accepted as true by those who seek for and obtain them, come just as religions do by revelation through intermediaries and are attested by miracles; revelations as good as any, and miracles as good as any. But, there being as yet no Church to declare which accounts shall be received as authoritative and which rejected as not, the Spiritualists find themselves encumbered with thousands of conflicting revelations. To be sure, these ought not to be held to the strict rules that apply where it is something

79

claimed to be the word of God that is to be judged, for they claim to be nothing more than words of deceased men, but it certainly is not unfair to criticise them by the same canons by which human testimony in earth-life is tested, according to which canons circumstantial details, in themselves insignificant, have their importance as criteria by which to judge the knowledge or veracity of a witness. Here are some of the most important contradictions to be found in the revelations in question:

There is a God. There is no God.

There is one only true devil. There is no devil at all. There is eternal punishment. There is only temporal punishment. There is no punishment at all; only infinite progression in wisdom and goodness. There is no pre-natal existence. We have passed through many earthly existences and must pass through many more yet, in order to learn on earth how to behave in heaven. These re-incarnations are for the gaining of experiences only. They are for experience and also for expiation of sin through suffering, i. e., for punishment. The Christian Bible is the word of God and is infallible. It is not the word of God, but only words of prophets under control of spirits of the dead and is fallible. There is no such place as hell. There is a perfectly orthodox hell, manned by devils quite scriptural. The occupations of the people of the spirit-world are like those they followed in this. They are not, but are quite different. There is a first, a second, a third and a fourth spiritual sphere. There are seven such spheres. There is only one. There is an indefinite number of them. This religion is the true one. That religion is the true one. No religion is true. The excuse for these conflicting stories is that they are colored by the beliefs of the medium or of the enquirers, or of the spirits invoked. But are the differences in them just shown, and for the correct giving of which every Spiritualist's experience may be referred to, differences of color? God and no God, hell and no hell, Bible and no Bible?

It is quite otherwise with respect to spiritual guidance in mundane affairs.

If the spirits engaged in such good work are the same as those who have for fifty years been trying to tell us something about the world they say lies next to this without as yet giving us a key-hole glimpse of it, then for their bad work in this latter respect they cannot be excused on the ground of stupidity, for in such guidance they give proof of having more than mundane wisdom, at least. If they are the same we have in them a source of information claiming to cover two worlds, that is to say, this one which they claim to have left and that one which they claim to have gone to, that tells us about that nothing we can believe and about this more than we ourselves know, just as if missionaries sent out to the heathen should be able to instruct them truly in all things relating to their own country, but be unable to tell anything but lies about that from which they were themselves sent. The proofs are abundant and incontestable that in countless cases there have come from intelligences claiming to be spirits of the departed instructions, warnings and predictions to guide and protect the living ; that from the same intelligences have come eloquent and wise discourses, theological, metaphysical, psychological and ethical, and not a few scientific and industrial discoveries and inventions ; that by them disease has been discovered and cured and calamities averted. In all which is abundant proof of love, benevolence, kindness, and watchful care, with desire to benefit mankind in every way. Why should beings truthful, intelligent, strong and good in relation to mundane things, pretend to a knowledge of things celestial that they are not possessed of, or conceal if they are ?

To be more specific, contradictions and absurdities in relation to matters and things of every-day life in the spiritual world that ought to be as well known to spirits dwelling there as the like things are to us here will be considered now under the heads of Dwellings, Clothing, Food, Locomotion and Occupations.

Dwellings in the Spiritual World

In the year 1883, a book entitled "Our Homes and Our Employments Hereafter", was published by Doctor M. Peebles, a well-known writer on Spiritualism, expressly to satisfy the demand for details of the spiritual world. "Give us details", his preface begins, "details and accurate delineations of life in the spirit world! — is the constant appeal of thoughtful minds. Death is approaching. Whither — oh, whither? Shall I know my friends beyond the tomb ? Will they know me ? What is their present condition and what their occupations ? " The work is chiefly made up of what are evidently the most rational and plausible "communications" the author could select, to the number of one hundred in all, and which are confessedly somewhat edited, in the interest of harmony of course. In respect to the most important detail, the sort of home to be found over there, and how acquired, we have on page 91 : " Spirits do not construct buildings from spirit substance by will-power alone. Mechanical skill and well-directed energies are required in the construction of machines, buildings and towering temples". On page 182 we have: "My house corresponds with what you call a dwelling, with its necessary surroundings. The labor of the hands, directed by cultivated taste and skill — intelligent will-power — were brought into requisition for its construction. I assisted in the building. Co-operation is the rule with us in such labors". But on page 128 is: " During our sojourn on earth our homes are prepared for us by the angels, and are built of the vibrations which go forth into the spiritual atmosphere from our hearts and lives. Will power, when it subdues evil, beautifies our home. When a spirit habitation is no longer required the atoms of which it is composed are dissipated, the spirits carrying with them up to a higher sphere the materials, which then form the nucleus of a more glorious home. Spirits who have gained a complete victory over matter can cause habitations to spring into being at will; and then they cease to exist as soon as no longer needed". If we have in this last an implication that though some spirits can build houses without hand-work, others have to ply the trowel or carry the hod, there is consolation in finding in another account that a little labor goes a great ways up there. On page 207 is: "The construction of homes in the spirit world of which I am an inhabitant does not require so much muscular effort as it does desire and will", and on page 166: "Once I saw a large company of spirits erecting a capacious stone building. It surprised me. I observed them until one story was accomplished, for they worked very rapidly". But on page 194, where a home is described as "studded with precious gems, with streams of water rippling over beds of diamonds and pearls, gardens containing every kind of luscious fruits", we further read that it was "not made with hands, but by the pure thoughts and good actions expressed in the earthly life". On page 212 is: "I found this home ready for me on leaving the earthly body. The silent work of construction went steadily on from my very youth on earth, and is still being carried forward, each act producing a corresponding effect on the structure". And on the same page the spirit of Horace Greeley says: "I have a home, lovely and grand — a home of nature's beauties, works of art, and gems of spirit literature — a located and real home — a home that increases in beauty as I progress towards eternal light — a home of which, during my earthly life, I was the unconscious architect and builder". Then he speaks of his wrong-doing and missteps, evidently alluding to his accepting the Democratic party's nomination for President. On page 224 is: " My home in my present sphere is ever made by myself, and not by another for me. It is truly a home not made with hands". In the Sixth sphere, as is stated on page 75, "they do not seem to have fixed habitations, but when they need a covering it is immediately improvised from the elements". In other places the dwellings, generally described as magnificent, are said to be " given by God", "prepared by the spirit", etc. But when the spirit of the intelligent A. A. Ballou speaks by the mouth of the brilliant improvisatrice and orator, Cora L. V. Richmond, we are told that there is really no need of house or home at all over there, and that in fact the only things that can be likened to them are but states. Thus, on page 219 is the following: " 'A house not made with hands, eternal in the heavens.' This quotation best describes a spirit habitation. Locality with reference to the astronomical or atmospheric condition is not essential. The house or home of the spirit must be essentially composed of the substance surrounding the spirit, and must be in the locality of the spirit's usefulness or labor. As heat and cold, winter and summer, poverty and riches, starvation and excess, changes of every physical kind, have no effect upon the spirit ; as the spirit does not require to be protected against the sun's rays or the wintry frosts and tempests; so our habitations are composed of just such substances, and are in just such localities as our spiritual necessities demand. What are those? Activity, The mind never sleeps; the spirit never ceases to act. Therefore we are not in need of a fixed habitation where we shall lay off the burthens of material cares, and rest or sleep as mortals do. I speak only for myself. Another of our spiritual necessities is the existence and presence of those for whom we have an affection. Our habitations, therefore, are largely our affections. We live in those ; they form the atmosphere surrounding us. That atmosphere takes shape of beauty, of variety, of light and shade, of architectural proportion, of art, of color, of line of form, according to our affections. Whatever there is of edifice or picture, of art or landscape in the atmosphere of our home, is the result of our lives, of our endeavor, of the action and thought that makes up our existence". On page 221 the same spirit continues: " In other words, to bring this statement within a compact and comprehensive form, that existence called objective on earth has no reality in spirit life". In which is flatly contradicted John Knowles, who, on page 196, says: "spirit homes are as much objective and as substantially real as are yours to you, while that existence called subjective on earth is the objective in spirit". "Houses and lands, gardens and flowers, organic life in every variety become the subjective with us. We have them if our affections require them; we have them not if our thoughts are beyond, or engaged in other directions". "There is no organic growth, animal or vegetable life, in high spiritual existence. By organic I mean generic physical growth. Every form of beauty, every bird, tree, flower, landscape, temple, is the result of some immediate action of mind, or intelligence, upon the atmosphere; and upon the particles composing that atmosphere of spirit life are the living pictures of the minds inhabiting that existence. They are not of themselves separate and apart from human entities as birds and flowers and trees are on earth, seeming to exist, whether man ever beheld them or not". But another authority, on page 245, comes to Mr. Ballou's support as follows: "Neither do we perceive any heat from the fire, or any cold from the frost". Another still, an English physician, on page 138, says : "We have no vicissitudes of climate, no uncleanness, no noxious insects or animals, no fear of thieves. We have no need of fires, nor do we require to cook our food. Other spirits on lower planes may". On page 176 is a description of the home of King Edgar Atheling, which reads: "There do not seem to be any places set apart for sleeping or eating; the first being to them a dreamy reverie, and their substance mainly derived from inhalation, of which the refuse is cast off through the pores of the skin by insensible excretion". Elsewhere another tells that spirits do not sleep. To sum up: dwellings in the spiritual world are, made by mechanical work, and not from spirit substance by will-power (this according to two accounts) — are prepared by the angels for us while we live — spring into being at will — when built by hand-work go up so rapidly that the labor must amount to nothing, — are not made with hands, but by pure thoughts and good actions — are made unconsciously by those who are to occupy them, while yet in earth-life, and, again, are truly homes not made with hands — are given by God — are " prepared " by the spirit — are not needed at all, since weather cannot affect a spirit, unless it be to represent his states — are subjective, and not objective, that is to say, are mere mental phenomena, as homes on earth are not.

Notwithstanding what is said to the contrary we are free to believe that no expenditure of labor is needed in the construction of the homes, since, according to one witness, hand-work is miraculously effective, running up a story of a large building while a passer-by stops to look on, and according to another, some spirits have such control over matter as to be able to create a house by a mere wish, and these will surely never refuse to build houses for others not so endowed. It must be a pleasure for them to do so, and as easy as for earthlings to blow soap-bubbles.

Clothing

That the reader may judge if the stories told of the clothes worn by spirits, their food, their occupations and modes of transporting passengers and freight are likely stories, and, incidentally, how far they agree one with another, here are given a few further quotations from Peebles, each quotation preceded by the number of its page. On page 62 we read: "In shape and appearance spiritual vestures correspond to the spirit's taste and custom when upon earth. The Quaker wears at first a plain dress. The Roman, the toga. The Oriental, the graceful robe. But in ethereality of texture, garments correspond to the moral States of the individual". 63 : "The first garments worn in spirit life are gifts of love. It is so with infants on earth. In the higher heavens robes and angel vestures are woven by will-power, through skilful hands, and woven almost in the twinkling of an eye". 92: "I saw a lady not long in the spirit life, engaged in needle-work. She had her spirit fabric of delicate texture, her spirit thread and needle. On earth she was a seamstress". 132: A Boston tailor is asked the question: "Was your external clothing prepared for you?" and answers: "It was, and brought to me and put on me, when I first escaped from the physical tenement". And to the question: " Did this spiritual clothing correspond to the spiritual status of your spiritual life?" he answered: "I afterwards perceived that it did, although I had no consciousness of this correspondence at the time". 140: "My spirit-clothing is the outgrowth of my mental states. It forms itself on my body, and is instantaneously in form according as my mind may vary its emotions, or frame of thought". "My clothing is of silk, velvet, lace, cloth of gold (or what would seem so to clairvoyants of earth), gauzy muslins, or simply white materials neither thick nor thin". "In the highest heavens angels are clothed upon with innocence, and are garmentless; but descending to lower spheres on acts of beneficence, appear clothed". "Will is the creator". 164: "Spirits that have just left their bodies appear clothed much as they were in their mortal form, while ancient and holier spirits are clad in celestial attire, shining as the sun". 173: "My garments were also prepared, and they corresponded with my taste, and, as I afterwards learned, with my moral status". 216: " My clothing was drapery ; I was conscious of that. It did not take the stereotyped form of earthly raiment; but I thought little of it, excepting that when a thought of delight pervaded the mind on each new recognition of a spirit friend, there would be a vibration throughout the whole frame which communicated itself to the drapery and to the atmosphere around me. That our friends are prepared to receive us in spirit life is certain; but spirit clothing, that which they adorn us with, that which is seen by many spirits (clairvoyants) in the form of raiment, is in reality their affections manifesting themselves upon the atmosphere that, like a shining light, surrounds us; and as our raiment is woven, not of material fabric, but of the aggregation of spiritual substances, so the thought and sympathy of our friends adorn us; we wear it as a shining raiment; atmosphere illumines and surrounds us; we are clothed in atmospheres". 260: " Our robes are the product of our lives, sadly, badly woven sometimes". Thus we see that spirits' clothing is sometimes the gift of love, sometimes woven by will-power, sometimes "prepared", how or by whom not being stated, is sometimes an outgrowth of mental states, taking form instantaneously, is sometimes nothing but the affections of the friends who bestow it, sometimes, in some way, the product of our moral deportment in earth-life, and, finally, in the case of angels, there is no clothing at all. Hand-work is hardly hinted at, and the conclusion must be that there is no work done on it of any kind, and the newly-arrived lady seamstress of page 92 was only doing a little repairing from force of habit. Except just after death, it is also plainly enough revealed that the clothing of each spirit is the expression of his character, thoughts and feelings, in short of his "states", which shows that Swedenborg's doctrine of correspondences is accepted by the spirits as to clothing as well as dwellings. In fact Swedenborg is often quoted by them, though sometimes with partial dissent, and it is stated in one place that he is installed as a teacher of spiritual analogy in some one of the spiritual spheres. In at least two places his affirmation that the spiritual world is a counterpart of the natural, is concurred in, notwithstanding both his spiritual world and that of these spirits are as different from the natural one as they are in most important respects from each other.

Locomotion

On this pretty important subject we have, page 141 : "A spirit may be conveyed with the rapidity almost of thought through space, according to the eagerness of his desire; or he may leisurely convey himself by walking, by floating, or by sailing on a boat; or, if on land, by a kind of carriage propelled by sails. All these modes of conveyance correspond to some frame of mind. Spirits are also seen upon horses and in chariots". On page 150 another account mentions "chariots, seemingly of fire", and also says: "elegant vehicles, drawn by horses and other kinds of graceful animals, here, as on earth, are subservient to the spirit's will". Another, on page 208, says: "There are gondolas, palanquins, carriages and chariots in my sphere of existence. Some would go from this place to London in half an hour; others would go almost like the lightning's flash". On page 72 mention is made of lakes with vessels and ponds with boats on them, also of boats that ply backwards and forwards, on the lakes, and on page 73, that those of the Sixth sphere were " building boats of a singular structure", and that in the same exalted sphere "they arrange their houses in groups, and have a kind of railroad to go from one group to the other; moreover, that they "traverse the ether spaces in aerial cars". But quite the contrary of all this, the spirit of Mrs. Kiddle (the wife of a distinguished Spiritualist who, because he was a Spiritualist, was expelled from the chief control of the public schools of New York City, to the immense and immediate injury of schools, teachers and pupils), says, on page 260: "We need no vehicles since the Lord has given us almost unlimited motion". This last might account for the absence of steam vessels and excuse the omission of the locomotive from spiritual locomotion were it not for the sail boats, sail carriages, fiery chariots, common chariots, elegant vehicles drawn by horses and other graceful animals, gondolas, palanquins, aerial cars, etc., that are mentioned. Here, as where clothing and houses are described, the land and water vehicles sometimes used by spirits represent their states and by analogy may be supposed to come as emanations or as representing the moods for the time being of those who go in them, that is, as produced by the same will-power which enables them to go where they please quick as lightning without any conveyance. At any rate we may presume that carriagemaking and boat-building are carried on in the same easy and expeditious manner as clothes are made and houses erected, so that the production of them does not amount to an occupation. Nothing is said about transportation of freight or baggage, or commerce in any commodities; which suggests the subject of

Food

In the upper spheres the sustenance of the spirits is, page 176, " chiefly derived from inhalation, of which the refuse is cast off through the pores of the skin by insensible excretion "; also, page 75, in those high places and states food " is compounded out of the elements and from etherealized fluids", and on page 71 we have: "He saw spirits preparing spiritual food composed of spiritual elements and auras". Below those, we are told in numerous places, the food is melons and delicious fruits, heavenly manna and nuts. Nothing is said of any expenditure of labor in cultivating the fruits; they may grow wild, or in orchards and gardens, but the probabilities are in favor of will-power such as produces the dwellings and clothing, since we have thus far seen that spirits, like us in the flesh, will do no more work than they can help, and are told on page 136, that it is possible to produce a bower of flowers by that same power, and if flowers, then of course fruit. Certainly it is a happy arrangement, in the interest of idleness, to make melons, fruits and nuts serve for food, since they need cooking no more than we can suppose heavenly manna does. As to flesh, fish and fowl, they seem to be allowed the American Indians, but no others, nor are grains or vegetables of any kind anywhere mentioned. And what has just been said of food, as well as what went before relating to clothing, would show there is no need in spirit-land to transport either freight or baggage, and so the absence of railroads, steamboats and steamships from the list given of means of locomotion is accounted for.

Thus between old ancestor worship and modern Spiritualism there is this most important difference, that in the first the dead must be fed by the living, while in the other they feed themselves.

Occupations

Swedenborg, as we have seen, makes the general statement that angels and spirits are very busy. Just so Peebles' spirits report that they " are never idle", but carefully avoid giving any details of their employment, as, for instance, when on page i6i the question is directly put, "How do spirits occupy their time, and what are the leading loves in your sphere ?" a Quaker tells how his brother painted pictures to decorate the walls of a house (was not Quaker Benjamin West turned out of the church for painting pictures?), and tells absolutely nothing more, neither concerning how spirits occupy their time, nor what are their leading loves, in a long answer that covers two pages octavo. And to this even more searching interrogatory, page 91 : " You deal too much, — pardon me, — in generalities. Be more pointed; tell me of one scene you have observed — one act that you have done to-day as a spirit?" All the reply that came was

87

what has been before substantially quoted concerning the spirit seamstress, and her spiritual needle and thread. A book made up of carefully selected revelations and that bears on its cover the title, " Our homes and our employments hereafter", and the first words of whose preface are: "Give us details" — quite omits, save in the two very small ones just quoted, any account of anything that will answer to the term industry. Houses, clothes, vehicles and food come without it. All industrial occupation being absent, what then are " our employments hereafter", of which revelations in detail are promised in the one hundred communications tendered by Dr. Peebles? In his summarizing Chapter 21, headed "The general teachings of the spirits", he himself quite forgets through all its sixteen octavo pages to even name houses, clothes, food, locomotion or any industrial occupations, such as keep men out of mischief in the natural world, or to give any hint of labor performed, save what is contained in two brief passages on page 279, which read thus: " They teach that the life of the spirits enter on after death is a sphere of struggle and moral conquest" — " that every moral altitude attained is a victory for the soul, purchased by self-denial, by aspiration, by persistent effort, and holy endeavor". " They teach that spirit life is an active life, a progressive life, with schools and lyceums, and museums and universities".

These generalities the reader of the book is allowed to fill in with such details as his imagination may supply, and he is also left to conjecture as he can how far the only occupations the spirits specify, namely, rearing children, instructing the ignorant, reforming the wicked and guarding mortals on earth, can fill up the time, or rather the eternity, of the vast population. It looks as if those whom Peebles in his preface implored to "give details and not generalities and vain imaginings", had so successfully befogged the subject and him as to make him quite lose sight of the object of his book, and left him to wind up with a mere gush of religionism unwarranted by the context. How is it that whatever revelation, biblical or other, has been given as coming from another world has been minute enough in respect to things of this one, as to morality, ritual, economics, proprieties, and even as to architecture, vestments and interior decoration, but vague unto nothingness as to what is and what is done in that other — voluminous and specific as to what we are familiar with; blank as to what we are not?

In effect the spiritual world of our Spiritualists, like that of Swedenborg's, is a world of idlers. In the case of mere bodiless souls there would be no question of tediousness, and the problem how such immortals could kill time need not trouble us. But in these spiritual worlds the inhabitants are complete and entire men, beings contrived for labor, whose life here chiefly consists in working for the means to live it. Nature abhors inaction, as she does any other vacuity. Human nature as we know it would render a heaven full of idlers a thing beyond imagining and only dreamable by a tired worker here below while his fatigue is on. It is impossible that such should be a happy world.

For the manifold errors, omissions, inconsistencies and contradictions in the volume of Dr. Peebles contained he seems to have seen the need of something of excuse or palliation, and at the close of his work, page 277, gives the best he can, which is as follows: "Just imagine several diverse characters reaching our shores from London, for the purpose of instructing us in the realities — the shame and the glory of London life. These shall embody patricians and plebeians, prince and peasant, judge and criminal, schoolman, tyro, scientist and shop-keeper, and other types of castes and conditions. It is plain enough that these persons, seeing London with different eyes, and while perhaps strictly honest would strangely differ in their descriptions. What would the novice know of the poet's library? And what conception could the poor day-toiler give us of the international questions often discussed in Parliament, or in the private councils of court life? And yet each of these characters would give substantially the same description of those features of London life accessible to common observation — such as the parks and gardens, the course of the Thames,

the dust and the fogs during certain seasons. And so spirits agree in regard to the general verities pertaining to spirit life — agree that there are landscapes and flowers, trees and running streams, houses and gardens, magnificent mountains and dismal lowlands, libraries and pictures, sympathies and antipathies, joys and sufferings, harmony and jarring discords". But the hundred selected spirits by no means substantially agree about anything, but disagree as widely as the Londoners would if they described their city as being built by will-power — not by will-power — of spirit substance — not of spirit substance — by vibrations which" go forth into the atmosphere from hearts and lives — by will-power of the kind that subdues evil — by people who have gained so complete a victory over matter that they can cause habitations to spring

up at will, which afterwards, when no longer needed, cease to exist — by hand-work, but of so expert a kind that a whole story of a large building is run up while a passer-by stops to look on — not by hand, but by pure thoughts and good actions — somehow constructed while its citizens were in process of gestation, so as to be ready for them as soon as they were born — local and real, but built by its inhabitants unconsciously to themselves — or of a given house as — not made with hands, but by the owner himself in some way kept to himself — not local at all, but coming at need to any locality — immediately improvised from the elements — not built at all, but given by God — prepared by the spirits — not needed at all, nor having locality, — made out of a sort of atmosphere that emanates from the intended occupants and which takes shape according to their affections. It is the same selected body of witnesses who tell us, concerning the clothing of the spirits, that it too comes in all the different ways, and is of all the widely different materials and makes just stated. It is they too who, in telling how spirits accomplish locomotion in that world the counterpart of this, omit the rail and engine and say nothing of steamvessels, or of electrical motors.

CHAPTER XV - RELIGION IN GENERAL

This word of manifold definition may conveniently be taken as meaning the cultivation of relations with the supernatural, understanding by this last the hidden part of the natural. In early times and while as yet natural phenomena, such as the movements of heavenly bodies and the play of elemental forces, were little understood, these served as a basis for religion as much as those others the how and why of which remain still unknown, and which for convenience may be termed supernatural phenomena, until science shall enlarge her borders and take them into her domain, as they have always been in that of nature. They can be classed as objective or such as are perceived as being outside of the perceiver, and subjective or such as are perceived as being within him.

Objective phenomena are the apparition of the double and like appeals to the outer senses, such as seem to confirm and support ancestor worship, and are adapted to the lowest order of minds because adapted to all minds. Coming into evidence early they did their work early, with belief of soul and its immortality as result. The like objective phenomena served to support beliefs in the lower order of gods.

But to the conception of God that arose in the Chinese, Greek and Aryan minds in their best estate, neither natural nor supernatural phenomena of the objective sort could have been the support. Such support could have been no other than those subjective intuitions which come to the solitary sage or saint in contemplative quietude impossible in very rude times, and requiring a perfected language to formulate. Though the god thus coming into belief was in fact merely the first principle in nature, it has been often invested with mundane qualities rendering it an object of love and worship, which fitly enough belong to the anthropomorphic ones which preceded it, but hardly to a metaphysical conception, which it is, as instanced by the invocation of Marcus Aurelius to the World, running thus: "O world I love that which thou lovest. Give to me what thou wilt; take from me what thou wilt. Whatever pleases thee pleases me. All comes from thee; all is in thee ; all returns to thee".

This may be because, although it is a purely philosophical conception, it did not come by the way of philosophy, but of revelation, that is of ecstatic intuition, Chinese, Hindu and Neoplatonic sages alike insisting on this, and declaring that such truth cannot be attained to either by books or study ; and thus coming it has the halo of supernatural illumination, forever accepted as guaranty of truth and forever inducing exaltation and fervor. Now such ecstatic intuition is as much a miracle as a spectre is, and thus the latest stage in religious evolution, belief in a philosophical god, like the first stage, belief in an immortal soul, has been attained through supernatural experiences; and these experiences being themselves actualities, whether truly or erroneously interpreted, religion has a basis of fact, therefore a scientific basis, and we need not look for such in any vague longings of the human heart arising none knows how.

The supernatural experiences in question having been everywhere the same, the various religions of the world may fairly be considered as having spontaneously arisen each on its own ground, save where the contrary is proved, or is fairly deducible, in the case of a given rite or dogma. The arising of modern Spiritualism in America and other countries where nothing was known of ancestor worship, is a case of a spontaneously originating, or reoriginating cult, Spiritualism being, as said before, precisely arcestor worship with sacrifice omitted.

Beliefs, Natural and Institutional

God and soul having thus established themselves in human belief, human ingenuity, stirred by human motives, set to work to build on it. Here is the province of speculation, fabrication, creed and ritual, orthodoxy, authority and priest-craft, in fine, of the Church. Ancestor worship, simple in its origin and by virtue of its simplicity able to do without priest or Church, has through all changes in other things kept its original character. And so, too, when the Hindu sets about finding his one only god and by junction with it obtaining release from re-birth, he goes to the woods and not to the temple, and there all by himself and for himself works out his own salvation; and obtains with that release, liberation also from all religious observance whatever, even from caste. And despite the efforts of the priesthood to envelop and absorb saints and sages and appropriate their merit, yoga practice under whatever name or guise remains essentially the same it always was. Should every religion that to-day exists disappear to-morrow and be lost from memory too, yet from elements inherent in the nature of man, he will again evolve a soul and a god, some sort of a god and some mode of immortality, and human nature remaining no better than hitherto, religions of widely varying sorts will arise again from these.

Subjective yoga is at this very time re-originating in America, as objective ancestor worship did a half century ago. Neither of them have needed to be imported; and both are plainly now the same they always were, as to phenomena. The doubles seen in ancient Egypt and the ghosts many times chased and sometimes found by the Society of Psychic Research of modern London are essentially alike. And the method by which the Patriarch Isaac "meditating at twilight" got his instructions from Jehovah, that by which the Hindu hermit attains to conscious one-ness with

Brahman, and that by which the possible " healer " now seeks development were and are one and the same, namely, mental concentration. The subjective phenomena equally with the objective are obtainable at first hand, and in their presence man stands as near to the supernatural — to the unknown causes of known effects — as is possible to him; all that comes after these is structure of his own fabrication.

The evolution of religious ideas has ever been hampered and hoppled by the dogma pervading all religions which accords the highest authority to the oldest revelations, compelling Hindu innovators to make their improved doctrines conform to the Upanishads and Vedic hymns, and Christian reformers to follow literally the whole Bible from Genesis to Revelations, or else wrest and wrench its meaning to their purpose. The result of thus chaining modern wisdom to ancient ignorance has given theologians a world of trouble, but the way in which those of India contrived to adapt the old ancestor worship which the people would not give up, and which, with its supernatural backing, would not let itself be given up, is a specimen of skill worthy of applause in any ecumenical council. Ancestor worship in its primitive form has no other destiny for the soul after death than the world of spirits. This was simple enough, but when the doctrine of reincarnation came to prevail the sojourn in that world had to be interrupted from time to time to permit of returns to earth; subject to such interruptions, the sojourn was perpetual, and the spiritual world still remained the final home of man. But later, and when it was discovered that that final home was to be in the bosom of Brahman, that re-incarnation was an evil, because all earthly existence was evil, and wise Hindus began to seek release from it through yoga practice, the old and new beliefs were seen to be altogether incompatible. To escape from these inconsistencies — to reconcile so they could live together the three doctrines of uninterrupted life in a world of spirits, life there interrupted by occasional returns to earth, and reabsorption in the creative principle — the term of sojourn in that world was cut short by definite limitations and the world itself divided into two, the one being, as before has been mentioned, the land of the fathers where the soul of a good man went on a vacation accorded as a reward of merit acquired by religious observances and good deeds to his fellows, for a term of time proportioned to that merit, to end in another re-incarnation, and the other being the land of the gods, attainable by yoga practice which had failed to carry the practicer quite up to Brahman, so that when, as was often the case, death overtook him while he was incompletely developed, and yet was too much a god to come back to earth again as a man. To suit such cases the other part of the world of spirits was appropriated to the use of such demi-gods demi-men, where they could tarry and resume and carry on to completion the work of self-deliverance. Thus adroitly was ineradicable ancestor worship not only reconciled with re-incarnation and its attendant Karma and with Yoga, but made to serve the uses of each.

This toleration by Hinduism in its perfected state of the primeval ancestor worship in which it had birth is justified by excellent results in moral guidance and spiritual comfort for the body of the people, but even if not by these, by the fact that having a scientific basis in those mystical phenomena so easily obtainable by all, it could not have been suppressed by any such means as Hinduism's tolerant spirit would have allowed it to take. Of course a like justification avails for all other religions, that have tolerated it. Again Hinduism stands acquitted of absurdity in respect to the retention in its celestial pantheon of myriads of gods old and new, and in its earthly temples of the myriads of idols representing them, as well as in respect to the enormous accumulation of rites and teachings regarding them, when it avows that all are but educational means for conducting ignorant but devout believers along a path that may in time bring them to something better — may conduct them by the way of religion out of religion and into a knowledge that dispenses with religion.

Hell

Every creed, however mild in the beginning, comes at last to have a hell, but it is said by those wise in such things that it is in every case a late comer. At first the threatening of mild and temporary punishments such as poor crops and barren cattle sufficed, but when later it became evident that such punishment by no means followed promptly nor certainly, upon transgressions, there happened what always happens when the execution of any law is neither summary nor sure; and the lawmakers resorted to severity as a remedy for uncertainty. But it is a remedy that must be forever ineffectual, save to make matters worse, and multiplying offences are again followed by increasing severity, for gods, priests nor any tyrants like to be frustrated, until at last offenders are no longer let off with sufferings which are merely incidental afflictions of their earthly life intensified, but are gathered together in some place where they can be systematically tormented; and this is hell, moderate and temporary at first, but in most cases getting worse and worse until it is roasting hot and eternally enduring.

The steps by which such a result is reached are well shown in the Chinese "Book of Rewards and Punishments. " It begins with implicitly recognizing the uncertainty and consequent inefficacy of the milder modes of discipline, by giving a series of accounts of cases wherein evil-doing had actually been followed by loss of health, wealth, life and especially of official position, in one generation if not in another, all very specific and in detail, with names, places and dates, so that any doubter might go and verify the statements. But after adding one earthly affliction to another, until every kind of mortal misery was appropriated as penalty for sin, it seems to have been found necessary to follow the sinful soul beyond the gates of death and punish it there in the way most appropriate to souls, namely, by making it pass through bodies of beasts, and that failing, through those of demons. Then, following the failure of even these, came imprisonment in Hell. Then Hell, having exhausted its terrors in vain, the whole series of inflictions that preceded it were added to it in one comprehensive cumulative sentence, and every torment bodies or souls could suffer, or gods or priests contrive, was hurled at sin. Could anything more be done to make men good? Yes; the children of the offender could, in case of earthly punishment, be included in the sentence to augment its intensity, and it could be inflicted on them alone in case he escaped, to increase its certainty of hitting somewhere. And this was accordingly done, and in China to-day the Divine law in this respect reads the same as that delivered to the Jews, and to which Christianity is indebted for its dogma of original sin. But in the book of rewards and punishments, it is only the worst grade of sinners that such clumsy justice applies to, as it is only the lowest of the populace who believe in and fear it; other grades it visits according to the measure of their" offences. So, also, did the Egyptian High Court of Assessors, with its weights and scales, and terms of transmigration of adjusted length, and a court open night and day, like the Court of Chancery, that there might be no delay of justice. So, also, does the Hindu Karma, which so operates that the exact penalty due every sin comes automatically and affixes itself and stays until full expiation is accomplished. Neoplatonism had very much the same method. And it is from this method of exactly adapting retribution to transgression that we have the word justice and not from indiscriminate, unmeasured, unweighed vengeance, as some people seem to think.

The mental attitude which most modern students of religion assume consists in turning the back on every supernatural occurrence or thing. Disporting themselves in the field of religious evolution, they ignore and pass by the most important class of religious facts, without which religion would be an altogether different thing from what it now is. Now, whether wisely or unwisely, the original religion makers believed in the supernatural, or at least adapted their work to the minds of those who did, and their thinking processes can hardly be comprehended by writers, however learned and acute, who not only disbelieve in it with all the energy of their nature, but wholly ignore the effect of belief in it on others. Thus Emile Burnouf attributes the conversion of Saint Paul to the remorse that came over him after assisting at the cruel murder of Saint Stephen, without even hinting at the account Paul himself gave of it when speaking for himself before King Agrippa, namely, a noonday vision, in which, surrounded with a light above the brightness of the sun, that caused him and his companions to fall to the earth, a voice spoke to and reproached him for persecuting

Christians, urged him to repent and do works meet for repentance, and concluded by telling him where to go and get initiated in the mysteries of Christianity. Other theorizers, in tracing out the evolution of the idea of one only god of the universe, write as if they never had heard of his having come to any meditating saint or yogi, in his ecstasy, filling him with light and joy and a conviction of divine reality and presence too absolute to be compassed by the word "revelation", or ever heard of the myriads of such who have in all times spent their lives in seeking God by solitary meditation, and believed they found Him with a faith that had all the force of absolute knowledge. And our theorizers write out their conclusions quite as if the idea in question could have come in no other way than the ordinary channels of thought and by dint of pure ratiocination.

The interpretation of the objective supernatural facts as meaning the immortality of the soul and the interpretation of subjective ones as meaning God, that have been heretofore made, may both of them fail, and yet supernaturalism in the end, and by the light of better investigation than has yet been given it, may be found to prove both God and immortality, though of a kind not hitherto conceived of, or it may be found to prove no such thing as either. The world is not yet so old but that its thinkers may be accused of making mistakes. And we of these times are quite at liberty to consider whether either group of supernatural phenomena has delivered its real message to mankind, and its last.

Morality and Religion

Morality, like hell, which is sometimes supposed to be its foundation, is also a late-comer into religions, and into more than one of them has never got at all. The gods of old Chaldea expended their wrath freely on offenders against themselves, and had little or none left for offences of man against man, that is to say, against morality. The Shinto, as we have seen, has no moral code. The Christian scheme of salvation in its original conception was a scheme for saving offenders from merited punishment, in itself an immoral proceeding. The sin charged up against all the children of Adam on account of an act of disobedience so transcendently grand as to merit the perpetual roasting with fire of one and all of them belittles into nothingness whatever they may commit against each other on their own account, and so belittles morality. It is true that Jesus taught a morality claimed to be as good as any prevailing in his time, and that the Ten Commandments are good so far as they go, but obedience to them both in every iota would not carry a man one step nearer to heaven or further from hell than the vilest sinner in the world, however much homilies and catechisms may insist on good works as an ornamental accomplishment. It is also true that after a few centuries of experience had shown the demoralizing effect of such a state of belief, the Church of Rome invented a purgatory, which it has never attempted to describe, much less to furnish plans and specifications of, and which fits so badly into the system it was added to as to make an incomprehensible muddle of what was before at least simple enough. Luther saved his church from such an incongruity by leaving out of it both purgatory and morality. According to Swedenborg he omitted good works and introduced justification by faith instead, because he would not imitate the Church of Rome which had lugged in good works late in time, to save a falling cause. Protestantism remains still without a morality, however moral Protestantdom may be. As a religion it lends no sanction of punishment or reward to the enforcement of good conduct on the earth, because the best man that treads it must go to hell unless he accepts Christ's offer of salvation, and the worst will go to heaven if he does. Logically, its concern is with Adam's immorality, and not that of his descendants.

Old Taoism never had a morality any more than it had a god. Chuang-Tzu in his exposition of it makes unceasing war upon Confucius, the greatest of the world's moralizers, and persistently sneers at his "charity and duty to the neighbor". Taoism declared for the "natural goodness of the heart of man", and for almost nihilistic freedom of human action. It was a high magic, and planed far above all terrestrial manners and customs; even virtue, humanity and justice were left below it. Its aim was goodness, to which all these were but the fallible means, and happiness was contained in that goodness. Beyond question, the Tao-Te-King sets up as high a standard of human conduct as any sacred book extant.

Finally, the gentle Eskimo, the best man in the world, is as godless and lawless as he is good.

Religion and morality ought never to have been associated. Each has been a disturber of the other. They cannot keep step together. Religion is in principle infallible, therefore unchangeable, therefore rigid, fixed, unshrinkable and unexpansive. Morality (manners) and ethics (customs) by their very natures are things of times and modes, of growth, and not of institution, and need room, time and freedom to grow. Religion does change, it is true, but since its principles are against change it hardly ever does so voluntarily, and usually has to be improved in the way despotisms are, by heresy and schism, corresponding to rebellion and revolution. Thus its modifications are painful and late-coming. And they have generally been forced upon it by growing morality that it had enveloped and closed, but could not forever hold hide-bound. During the last half century American Protestantism has been amended by the addition of two new sins, namely, holding slaves and drinking wine, both undoubtedly sanctioned by the Bible as much now as ever, as distinctly as eating meat is, which great efforts are being made to degrade in its turn into the category of sins. But the contest over these questions, in which the defenders of the Bible have been clearly in the right, has so wrenched and shaken its authority in the estimation of people that it remains to-day too weak to effectively maintain a single point of doctrine after it has gone out of fashion as a point of morality.

It would be wrong to say that the sanctions afforded by religion to morality are ineffective, but in making a nursling of anything it is also made a weakling; and Christianity, having in course of time become discredited, the morality of Christendom, bereft of its prop, has, no doubt, suffered in many respects, notably in honesty. But to countervail this, the gain has been so great in humanity and tolerance, kindliness and charity, that a considerable profit remains from the decadence of faith; while there also remains a fair inference that the natural evolution of society, liberated in part by that decadence, has in all respects done better work than before.

That morality should be left free to achieve progress on its own account and go its own way towards its own evolutionary goal is the more evident when it is considered how very remote that goal still is. The time is yet far off when the natural tendency which Spencer has well shown altruism has to run itself out shall bring in a social state wherein every man will be so bent on doing good to others that the only injury others can possibly inflict on him will be to refuse to let him do it. If we are thus remote from the attainment of ideals presently existing, much more so must we be from that which the Tao-Te-King affirms to have existed in ancient China, and beyond which it seems inconceivable that any ideal could go. According to that, the Chinese race at least once actually enjoyed and afterwards fell from a social state that was above virtue, above humanity, above justice, thus above morality — a state wherein each man did virtuous acts without dreaming he had virtue, and humane acts without dreaming he was humane, and only when he had so far back-slidden as to be simply just did he know that he was so. Turning and looking back toward such a golden age, real or supposed, wherein not even a golden rule was needed for man's guidance, nor anything like religion known, and setting before the mind the ideal from which one people are said to have fallen as the one to be aimed at by all, those of our day may easily see that in running the race set before her morality will make the better speed the less she is harnessed to religion or anything else.

Kant claimed to have found in the moral law, discoverable by conscience, and an inborn sense of obligation to follow it, the best imaginable guaranty of good conduct. He declared that one who by reference to that law was restrained from committing an evil action which otherwise he would by force of evil impulses within him have committed, was more praiseworthy than one who had no such impulses to restrain. If Kant in " Texts of Taoism" meant by this that praise and credit should be accorded as an encouragement to those who could or would do good only when that law required them to, and need not be bestowed on those who needed no such encouragement, he was right enough. But if he meant to say that these last were not more admiration-worthy and love-worthy, and more creditable to their Creator than the others — or meant to say that the perfect man of Lao-Tsee was not a more desirable citizen of the world than they, he was wrong. There is no man who would not rather travel round the globe with a companion who could feel no impulse, nor respond to any temptation to injure him, than with one whose heart continually prompted him to murder and rob, but who as continually resisted, however effectually, the prompting, because on second thoughts he recalled that there was a moral law within him which prohibited robbery and murder, and that to break it would make him feel more uncomfortable than to keep it. The object of Kant's praise must be ranked in the third degree of moral degradation, according to the classification of the Chinese sage, namely, in that of justice, requiring, to keep him in order, constant reference to law, and acting always "with intention " ; while those, if such now exist, in the degree next higher, humanity, or the next higher still, virtue, both being yet below the highest moral state, Tao, know nothing of intention, nor require to consult conscience, doing as they will, and not as they must.

CHAPTER XVI - THE EVOLUTION
OF SOCIAL VIRTUE

For the established fact that men's good dispositions toward each other are capable of improvement, and do improve by living together under orderly conditions, many causes have been supposed besides religion. First in order comes law, with force at its back, as in the case of governmental enactments, or with only moral sanctions of punishment or reward resting in public opinion and social esteem, or the expectation expressed in the saying of Lao-Tsee that "whatsoever you do unto others, that also will they do unto you". Out of long-continued obedience to law grows the habit of doing what it commands and also the notion that it is more the law we have to answer to than the principles it formulates, from which habit and notion has arisen the belief taught by Kant, but controverted by Schopenhauer, of a categorical imperative, a "must", an "ought", that every man is born with, impelling him to obey a moral law that is also his birthright; and from them too has also arisen the idea that justice, something incidental to and qualifying the application of a general law to particular cases, is the principle of morality.

Another and a potent cause is the extension of sympathy, love and friendship which close and long-continued relations of men with each other, fostered by peace and social order, tend to bring about. These softening influences originating in the family, thence extending to the tribe, thence to the neighborhood, and thence to the nation, finally reach out to the whole world — or at least such is their tendency. There was a time when the mating of the sexes brought with it no sexual love, but it came. There was a time when paternal love was a stranger to the human heart, but it came. There was a time too when all outside the tribe were enemies or prey, for whom in their sufferings no pity was felt, and in whose joy there was no rejoicing. If one kind of love can grow in the heart, and improve its dispositions to good, so can another, and another still; and all men may become brothers, and loving ones, if they will only keep the peace long enough. If for instance sexual love is a principle in man's nature, acting of its own motion, and independent of evolution, though capable of being developed by it, so may be all other love, whether arising between children of the same family, or reaching out to universal brotherhood.

Still another cause is by certain mystical philosophers found in sympathy. The knowledge which the unconscious part of us is by such supposed to have, that all mankind are one, so that when one strikes another he hits himself, they consider to be the true basis of morality. As such knowledge is only imparted to the consciousness through channels properly called intuitive, this doctrine commends itself to the intuitional school of moralists; while, seeing it resolves the motive to moral conduct into pure selfishness, it equally should commend itself to the opposite school of utilitarians, whose teachings the first opprobriously denounce as selfish. Much may be said in favor of the moralizing efficacy of this sub-consciousness of a transcendent unity. The foregoing are the most important of the theories advanced by those who labor in thought over the problem of ethical evolution. Probably most readers will judge that of all the causes above stated as working out that evolution, law and force are the worst, and sympathy and love the best. That these last are also the most efficient is of late coming to be recognized in pulpit-teaching, which yearly relies more on love and less and less on terror; though our law-makers, by the multiplicity of their enactments of late years so notable, show that they are far from having learned that all law is essentially evil, and only justifiable by strong necessity. But are there not still other causes at work to induce in men's natures dispositions to good conduct ?

The world did not have to wait for modern science to discover and proclaim the power of mind over mind by other and more direct means than logical ones, and the resulting control over the thought, will and actions of one person by the intentions of another. Nor was Plotinus telling news when in the second century after Christ he said: " Every being who has relations with another can be bewitched by it; it is bewitched or attracted by the being with which it is in rapport. It is only the being concentrated in itself (by contemplation of the intelligible world) that cannot be bewitched. Magic exerts its influence on all action and on all active life, for active life tends towards things which enchant it", But long before Plotinus wrote Chinese rulers actually applied the principle to the government of their states, calling in from their seclusion sages "concentrated in themselves " to bewitch bad citizens into becoming good ones. All know that cases are common of couples who begin their married life in a state of habitual strife, but who, as years go on, grow more and more peaceable, and finally close it as friends, if not as lovers — a result, to be sure, which may in a measure be due to their learning by experience to avoid causes of contention and contact with each other's rough points, but is sometimes so marked as to bring in the supposition that it may also be due to mutual, long-continued, unconsciously-exerted "suggestion" operating in their natures permanent changes of dispositions, a process as mysterious as that which, in couples who begin as lovers, brings them, at the end of a long and harmonious life, to look and think alike, something often noticed, admired and wondered at.

All which looks as if the supernatural sometimes comes into the province of familiar life to play its part as an evolutionary force, or at least something not usually credited with such power. Moved by self-interest, each member of a given community must desire that every other shall be good to him, which is the same as saying that all will desire that all others shall be kind, just and orderly, and so desiring, will in their business or social intercourse be continually influencing each other, by true hypnotic "suggestion", to altruistic acts. The buyer will habitually suggest to the seller to be content with moderate profits and give good measure, and the sick man will mentally implore the physician to nurse him and not the disease. And against the concentric suggestions of all who deal with or employ them, these will have no resisting power beyond the selfish desire and mental action of their respective selves — in each case it will be the auto-suggestion of one against the direct suggestions of many. The result will be more than a succession in each supposed case of altruistic acts which leave the inner nature of him who performs them untouched, a series of good deeds done, by a bad man it may be, under magical compulsion, for a hypnotized person acts from the immediate impulsion of his own subjective mind, which alone is amenable to control by suggestion, and his acts seem to him to come spontaneously from his own will. Therefore, the suggestion that he perform a certain neighborly duty is also a suggestion that he is a good neighbor, which by repetition tends to make him such in reality. Contrary to this would be the case of a slave, compelled by fear of the lash to do the same acts that such a neighbor would do from a good disposition. He would have his fears strengthened, but hardly his benevolence, by the discipline. Evidently those actions of man towards man which spring from fear of punishment or hope of reward must be in their essence external and leave the inner nature of him untouched ; whereas the quasi-hypnotic suggestion, by which the concentric selfish wills of a whole community act on the individual impulses of each, enters into the very nature of each and works a permanent change; and this, as said before, because every suggestion to do a good act is also a suggestion that it is to be done from a spontaneous impulse, and so amounts to a suggestion to be, naturally, and therefore permanently, good.

Human activities result from human nature acted on by earthly conditions. A superior nature may overcome evil conditions and an inferior nature may fail to react under good ones, but in all cases both elements have to be taken into account in reasoning from the past to the future. Is it possible that at any past epoch there has existed on our earth a race of men so highly favored in their inborn dispositions and outward circumstances that a social state has resulted, justly entitling that epoch to be called a golden age? Lao-Tsee insisted that there had, as indeed others of the ancients did, though none so emphatically as he ; and in his striving against the school of moralists, whose work was doubtless rendered necessary by the growing wickedness of his people, which he admitted, but would not admit could be cured by moralization, turned his face toward it as to an age himself had dwelt in (if not during his then lifetime of twelve hundred years, at least in some one of his earlier reincarnations), wherein men could keep order without law, do good to one another without religion, and be happy in their loves without morality, knowing, as he expressed it, their mothers but not their fathers — an age wherein good actions were spontaneous, and performed without reference to any rewards or punishments to follow, or even consciousness that they were virtuous, humane or just.

The totality of the orderly conditions which permit the evolution of goodness in the heart of man is summed up in the words security and freedom, and these again in the word peace. Egypt and Babylonia developed their civilization under the shelter from hostile invasion afforded by bordering deserts and seas. India, Greece and Italy are peninsulas sealed by mountain ranges. Britain and Japan are islands. But the happy society of the golden age to which Lao-Tsee has alluded, in the Tas-Te-King, if it ever existed, needed a far greater measure of tranquillity for its evolution than such civilization as we know of did. The people attaining to it, or born into it, must have been so averse to violence as to abstain from going to war, and also disposed and able to keep war from coming to them; moreover, able and disposed to live together in peace without need to invoke that other form of violence called law. But never in any age of the world would a people so constituted have been allowed to occupy any desirable territory, or in fact any part of the habitable globe, properly so called, while there were warlike races who coveted it; and pressed upon by such, the lovers of peace must have been driven from place to place, until a final refuge was found in a region uninhabitable by their pursuers. Such a region is the narrow belt which bounds on its southward limit the great ice-cap of the north, a belt which is now to be looked for in Alaska and Greenland, but which once was found as far southward as central France. This movable Arctic circle, so to call it, the refugees would be forced to follow, as with increasing warmth of climate it slowly moved northward, subsisting as they went on their fellow refugees the reindeer, mastodon and musk ox, or perishing by the way. And to subsist and not perish they must have been intelligent, vigorous and heroic.

On the American shores of the Arctic Ocean, hemmed in between perilous waters and frozen land, some forty thousand Eskimos yet manage to keep alive. They are of the type that has been termed mongoloid, though of much lighter complexion than the mongols proper, of stature averaging five feet, six inches ; well formed, hardy and strong and with agreeable and smiling faces. They are exceedingly intelligent and skillful, remarkably ingenious, with astonishing readiness in emergencies, learn rapidly, have much artistic skill, a taste for music, and a keen sense of humor. "Their invention and dexterity" are, according to Captain Cook, "at least equal to that of any other nation". Though strongly averse to war, yet when assailed by their savage neighbors, they fight fiercely and well, while in their habitual encounters with the turbulent sea and its monsters they show a heroism which proves that courage naturally and of right takes its place among the virtues in a perfect character, nor needs for its development the practice of man-slaying. In the Journal of the Ethnological Society for 1848, the characteristics of the Eskimos are summed up thus: "They are uniformly described as scrupulously honest, careful of the aged, affectionate to their children, devotedly attached to each other and fond of their domestic animals. So little are they inclined to quarrel that after two years' acquaintance with the natives of Melbourne Peninsula, Sir Edward Parry has related only one case where it extended to blows". It is further said of them that they share their food as a matter of course with whoever is in need. As a phrenologist would expect, their skulls are described as " largish " and also as high, showing a good development of the moral faculties. They are " morbidly anxious not to give offence", fastidiously ceremonious and polite, carrying the latter virtue so far that it is said, "They always, in their dealings with the Danes of Greenland, leave it to the buyer to fix the price of what they sell", and "in their intercourse with each other indulge in much hyperbolical compliment and language courteous from the teeth outward". Father Barnum, a Jesuit missionary lately from among them, adds his testimony to the foregoing by telling us they are gentle, hospitable and goodnatured. He also says their language is magnificent and rich, very complicated, and free from harsh sounds.

Per contra, though absolutely honest towards each other, it is said that some of them will sometimes steal "unconsidered trifles", like harpoons, fish-hooks, knives, etc., left in their way by strangers; but concerning this, Captain Parry truly observed: "We must make due allowance for the degree of temptation to which they were daily exposed, amidst the boundless stores of wealth which our ships appeared to them to furnish". They can bear grudges too, will secretly injure those who injure them, and will even lie in wait and kill an enemy; and "when a murder is committed it appears that the nearest relation or most intimate friend of the slain has a right to kill the murderer"; this is secretly, of course, for they are so averse to violence that they will "not even kill an enemy except by stealth. " This bearing grudges and secretly revenging injuries would naturally result from aversion to violence whether of words or deeds and depend on the same principle which causes them, good fighters as they are when pushed to the wall, to avoid war as long as they can; thus it is from a principle of mildness, itself a form of goodness, that they in such cases act. But such retaliations must needs be rare, and only resorted to in cases clearly proved, or they would not be acquiesced in by the community, and would besides bring on counter and cumulative retaliations, necessitating an established government. They are in reality judicial proceedings carried on without cost to the county. Lastly, the Eskimos are accused of sometimes indulging in polygamy and polyandry, and of tolerating without the least pang of jealousy the freekindness their wives manifest towards strangers. In short, although their family methods are such as are entirely to their own liking, they have not yet adopted ours. Let the most be made of this that can. And making the most of all the foregoing, and even allowing nothing for the prejudice of the missionaries through whom chiefly the accusations have come, nor for the contaminating contact of the Europeans and Americans, whose worst representatives have been for a century and more taking advantage of the afore-mentioned free-kindness to adulterate the Eskimo's blood with their own racial ferocity of character and poison it with syphilitic virus, while their best ones have been trying to make death terrible to them instead of what they have been used to consider it, a welcome relief from a life of peculiar hardships and an entrance into a paradise as good as they can imagine, there still remains a people whose conduct is sufficiently perfect for all practical purposes, a people in fact as much so as they could be and not be quite characterless. They are, literally speaking, too good for this world, since their best virtue, aversion to war, has disabled them to hold their own in any part of it of use to other races. "What an admirable government they must have had", one who holds morality to be a creation of statecraft might exclaim; "what severe laws, what a welldrilled police, what sharp detectives, what strong prisons, what frequent executions!" While one who traces moral evolution to a religious origin will say, " what a severe god, what a cruel devil, and what a hot hell must have been theirs!" But no; these good outcasts are absolutely without government, or law, God or religion, morality, or even customs. Like the Chinese of the golden age, they do good not because commanded to do so by any of these, nor because it is right, but because it is their humor to do so. "They have", says one authority, "no chiefs or political or military rulers". One Fabricius described them in his day, as " Sine Domino regunter, aut, consuetudine". " They live in a state of perfect freedom", says another, "no one apparently claiming authority over or acknowledging the least subordination to another except what is due from children to their parents; an Eskimo is subject to no man's control". It is true that they take counsel of their elders, by some travellers thought to be chiefs, and employ medicine men, by some mistaken for priests, but the former pretend to no authority and the latter do not undertake to rule the natural world from the spiritual one; " no kind of religious worship seems to exist among them", says one traveller, and Lubbock's " Pre-historic Times " quotes Crantz as saying: "The Greenland

Eskimos have neither religion nor idolatrous worship, nor so much as any ceremonies to be perceived tending towards it".

There is an old story of a sick king whom nothing could cure but wearing the shirt of a perfectly happy man; but unfortunately, the only perfectly happy man to be found in his whole realm never had owned a shirt. In like manner, were the modern rulers of a sick state to send commissioners to the good folk of Greenland or Alaska to obtain copies of their bible, statute book or moral code to apply to the healing of their nation, those commissioners would have to return empty-handed and report that the best race on the globe were absolutely without government, none of them ever intentionally obeying a law, or a "categorical imperative", keeping a commandment or following a custom, but that each did as he pleased because it pleased him to do so. They might also report that though the Eskimos believe themselves to be the happiest race on the earth and have much pity for all others, not one among them ever had a shirt to his back.

But they have in a large degree the virtue of being sensitive to public opinion. " Nothing so effectually restrains the Greenlander from vice as the dread of public disgrace, "says one authority. Another tells us: " They decide their quarrels by a match of singing and dancing which they call the Singing Combat. If a Greenlander thinks himself aggrieved by another, he discovers no symptom of revengeful designs, anger or vexation, but he composes a satirical poem, which he recites with singing and dancing in the presence of his domestics and particularly the female part of his family, till they know it by rote. He then in the face of the whole country challenges his antagonist to a satirical duel, ... he who has the last word wins the trial". Surely so mild a chastisement as this, and the knowledge that every serious trespass on the neighbor will bring a quietly and secretly inflicted retaliation in kind, the offence being the measure of its own punishment, would have advantages over the rule of brute force as Godwin calls it, on which civilized society relies to preserve order.

Kindred to, one might say identical with, their aversion to be governed is the dislike of the Eskimos to control of every kind. It is very difficult to induce them to enter into a contract of service, though when they do it is observed with "slavish" fidelity. They are the truest lovers of freedom that live. Their aversion to war, on which their destiny, and may be that of the whole human race has turned, is important enough to be well considered. Its roots must lie deep in their natures. One root may be their repugnance to the presence of death. The traveller Hall reports that "they have a superstitious objection to use, or even touch, anything that has been in a house containing a dead body". And they remove it for burial not by the door, but by a window, or if there be none, through a hole made for the purpose. From this repugnance, mingled with an extreme sensitiveness to the sufferings of others, especially of those they love, it is that in some cases "where a person is evidently dying they place by him everything which can soothe and comfort his last moments, including warm covering, and leave the ingloo or house, which they close up, thus converting it into a tomb".

Another root may be their sense of shame, a sense of no mean importance as a regulator of human conduct. (Schopenhauer goes so far as to say that where it arises it is good proof that the act which causes it is evil, procreation,for instance.) With the Eskimos war is indecent and murder obscene. Strange as it may seem, and hard as it may be to explain, to them, violence of every kind is something to blush for; and this being admitted, the power of mere shame to restrain from deeds of violence may easily be also admitted. The vestal virgins were withheld from suicide by knowing that if any of them should commit it her body would be publicly exposed. King Candulus had to die because he offended his wife's modesty by showing her naked to his friend. And if every senator and representative of ours who should vote to declare war were compelled to exhibit himself before the first army that marched to battle in like plight with that modest, murderous queen, unquestionably he would be thereby inclined to peaceful counsels.

Another root of this hatred of strife so strange in a world of slaughter like ours may be that evenness of temper often wondered at by all who go among the Eskimos. Just as great billows cannot rise and rage except the surface of the sea be first rippled with wavelets, and in fact depend on them, since when the wavelets are quieted with a little oil the billows subside, so human rage depends for its support on the irritability of men's tempers, and cannot arise while they remain unruffled. Now this support singularly fails in the case of the imperturable Eskimos, of whom Captain Lyon remarks "... that their evenness of temper is not surpassed, if equaled, by any other nation". Another observer goes further still, and Father Barnum relates that on one occasion he was in a boat manned by them when, just as it was being pulled past a most dangerous point, where it required the utmost care and steadiness to avoid being carried by a current upon and dashed against a point of rocks, one of the crew maladroitly broke his oar, and that in the season of suspense which followed and while the man was striving to pull forth another from the bottom of the boat and get it into position, he looked first at the rocks that seemed to roar louder for the prey that was nearing their jaws with every anxious instant that passed and then at the faces of the crew, but saw no sign nor heard any word of anger or impatience ; instead, only a smile of surprise ; nor was the offender reproached afterwards. A crew of Americans might have kept silence while the peril was upon them, but could they have smiled ? And would they not as soon as safe sworn with many oaths and much emphasis? Such a people could not easily be stirred to make mobs of themselves and shout "Nacht Paris .' " or " A Berlin ! " An imperturbable temper, is it not of like quality with the state of mental and emotional indifference which after years of tranquil contemplation comes to reward the Hindu yoga or other saint, and which Plotinus describes as so complete that a true sage, one who had "attained", could witness unmoved the sacking of a city; so that the word "philosophical" has in common parlance for one meaning, quietude of temper?

Retaliation in kind could not be practiced by any less philosophical people than the Eskimos, without resulting in a state of anarchy such as would make a government of some kind necessary. That it has not in their case may be attributed to an inertia of temper which only a much greater provocation than would suffice to stir ours can move to violence, and also to an altruism much surpassing ours. And we must suppose that in Greenland and Alaska the retaliatory punishment is justly proportional to the offense, and is therefore submitted to without bringing on counter retaliation as it would in so-called civilized countries, where accordingly it could not be allowed to take the place of law, though it often rages despite of law, especially in America, in some parts of which country the counter retaliation brought on by bountiful over-measure of revenge occasionally extends till it involves large family connections in feuds that become hereditary, and sometimes only end with the extermination of one of the warring clans.

In disputes between nations, each party being its own judge, is sure to overestimate its injuries and claims and underestimate those of the other, and in exacting redress or inflicting vengeance the one will be as sure to do so in over-measure and the other to refuse submission to it even if under-measured, and to cherish hopes of reprisal and re-revenge. Thus war breeds war, and a state of national anarchy has arisen like what would arise if in courts of justice each plaintiff in a proceeding were, besides drafting his complaint, to bring in his own verdict, render his own judgment upon it, and take the execution of that judgment into his own hands. To day Christendom on both sides of the ocean seems only pausing from battle to get its breath; and who but knows that the evolution of humane dispositions, which has of late achieved its best result in causing the British people to abandon private warfare in the form of duelling, must, operate a long while yet before that or any other people will allow its government to accept as the Eskimos must, and be content with, less than the full measure of redress it conceives itself entitled to have. Before private warfare could be brought to an end in the British Isles some one gentleman of high standing and known courage had to take an insult without giving a challenge. What great nation will begin the ending of national warfare by pocketing an insult or forgiving an injury ? A question out of which arises another: what ministry or party could keep in power after a vote to do either ? The few reflect, the multitude rage, and rage prevails.

The peaceful Eskimos, by choosing to run rather than fight, have secured for themselves, we may say, five thousand years of tranquillity during which the forces that make for altruism could work. Had they been allowed during those years to dwell in the temperate zone instead of being driven to the snows to live without fire or water, the fruits of their long peace might have been something more than the practice of social virtue among some widely scattered outcasts.

There can be little doubt that the remnant of forty thousand, which is all they now count, represent a much larger number who once found refuge in the larger belt of polar region accessible to them when the southern boundary of the ice-cap was traced across the central parts of Asia, Europe and America. Possibly the ancestors of the Eskimos may once have spread over large portions of the temperate zone, and afterwards been driven from it by warlike tribes multiplying upon their borders; a small pack of wolves can chase a large flock of sheep. It seems to be now the opinion of those who investigate such things that the cave-dwellers of Central Europe were of the same race as the present Eskimos. One authority tells us that: "These traces of the most ancient races of men as yet discovered in Europe may with a high degree of probability be referred to the Eskimos. The bone needles and many of the harpoons, as well as the flint spear-heads, arrow-heads and scrapers, are of precisely the same form as those now in use among the Eskimos. The artistic designs from the caves of France, Belgium and Switzerland are identical in plan and workmanship with those of the Eskimos, with this difference only, that the hunting scenes, familiar to the Palaeolithic cave-dwellers, were not the same as those familiar to the shores of the Arctic Ocean. Each represented the animals which he knew, and the whale, walrus and seal were unknown to the inland dwellers of Aquitaine, just as the mammoth, bison and wild horse are unknown to the Eskimos. The reindeer, which they both knew, is represented in the same way by both. The practice of accumulating large quantities of the bones of animals round their dwelling-places, and the habit of splitting the bones for the sake of the marrow, are the same in both. The hides were prepared with the same sort of instruments, and the needles with which they were sewn together are of the same pattern. In both there was the same disregard of sepulture. All these facts can hardly be mere coincidences caused by both people leading a savage life under similar conditions. The conclusion, therefore, seems inevitable that, so far as we have any evidence of the race to which the cave-dwellers belong, that evidence points only in the direction of the Eskimo" . . . "The reindeer and musk sheep afford food now to the Eskimos in the Arctic Circle, just as they afforded it to the Palaeolithic hunters in Europe; and both these animals have been traced by their remains from the Pyrenees to the northeast, through Europe and Asia as far as the very regions in which they now live. The mammoth and bison, too, have been tracked by their remains in the frozen river gravels through Siberia as far as the American side of the Straits of Behring. Palaeolithic man appeared in Europe with the Arctic mammalia, lived in Europe with them, and in all human probability retreated to the northeast with them." It will be noted that the course of the migration here set forth was through regions now included in the Chinese Empire. Could it have been that a portion of the on-moving lovers of peace halted and stood at bay, then turned on and overcame their pursuers, or by the exercise of their superior intelligence got control of the tribes pressing upon them just as the migrating Hindus mastered the aborigines of Hindustan, and just as the Chinese did, in fact, after the dawn of history, master those of the valley of the Yellow River into which they descended from the North ? Could it have been that ages before this descent they became in some such way masters of their own movements, then fusing more or less with their ferocious neighbors, became warlike enough to hold their own, and ceasing to be nomads, settled down as husband-men, and so became Chinese, while others, moving on, became the Eskimos, as we know them now ? Both the Chinese and Eskimos are Mongolian in type, both are of lighter complexion than others of that type, and both have narrow eyes, such as are supposed to result from snowglare in frozen regions, and such as even the animals who exist there show. Professor Tiele, of Leyden, writing under the heading of "Religion" in the Encyclopsedia Britannica, says the Eskimos have many of the Mongolian customs. They resemble the Chinese again in being excessively ceremonious and polite, preferring to lie rather than hurt the feelings of others, and in having great artistic ability and handicraft skill. The Eskimos dislike to be governed; the Chinese, though overmuch governed, dislike it, too; have as little as possible to do with courts or officials, and buy their peace of both with bribes, just as they would pay tribute to brigands. And the ability to do without government or law, which the Eskimos actually prove themselves to possess, was matched in the legendary China of Lao-Tsee, wherein men were good without regard to law, and whence seem to have come down to historic times strangely democratic, or rather nihilistic, ideas, which have found expression in sayings of their great sage like these: "He who rules ruins" ; "Let him rule the empire who can let things alone" ; " The more regulations the worse off the people" ; "The more show of penalties the more rogues, therefore the wise man says, I will be quiet and the people will have a chance to improve themselves" ; " Overlegislation increases crime"; "If the government is meddling there will be constant law-breaking". "The right of rebellion, "says one writer", enters into the very texture of Chinese education". Another calls them, "the least revolutionary, but the most rebellious of peoples". The

Chinese as known in historic times cannot be expected to prove their descent from the cave-dwellers by emulating the lawless goodness of the present Eskimos, seeing their history is that of a warlike people, and they have largely adulterated their blood with that of the ferocious tribes they have absorbed, both of which causes would have hindered the evolution or the practice of such goodness; yet they were good enough to have become a thousand years ago the most civilized people in the world, and seventeen hundred years ago Ptolemy could write of them that they were "civilized, mild, just and frugal", and to-day there can be no doubt in any informed and impartial mind that life and property are as safe among them as in any country on the globe, nor that in the conduct of their relations with other nations they have shown a better morality and humanity than Great Britain or the United States can boast. As in respect to the aversion to being governed we have to look for a parallel to Eskimo practice in Chinese precept, so in respect to the spontaneous goodness of the Eskimo we have to look for a parallel mainly to the Chinese ideal, as it has always been held to, and held to, be it noted, as an inheritance from prehistoric times, "At the base of the whole Shu King", says Samuel Johnson, " is the characteristic Chinese faith in an inherent moral sense in all men, whose sanctions are not found in fears of hell or hopes of heaven, and whose acknowledged origin in the nature of things leaves no room for arbitrary divine will". Again he says: "That morality does not depend on such separation of reason and faith (religious sanction) is clearly proved by the fact that no race in the world has attained by the habitual use of it to so pure an ethical consciousness as the Chinese have reached without it, and none, it is probable, on the whole, a practical conduct more free from the gross vices". And this tradition of the natural goodness of man has even infected the moralization of Confucius, so that his disciple Mencius sententiously expresses it in the saying: "Who knows his own nature knows heaven". That this high ideal of right conduct and of the natural goodness of the heart of man does not rest in idea merely, but is believed to actuate mankind at large, and their rulers, too, was well illustrated by the letter which the Imperial Commissioner Lin addressed to the Queen of England, in which he appealed directly to her heart and conscience not to force into the ports of China a drug poisonous to soul and body, using language that must have made her sigh with regret that the interests of trade and the limitations of the British Constitution restrained her from making other reply than with bullets and bombs, fire and blood. "How then", said he, " an you bear to seek gain by means of an article so injurious to man, and without compunction of conscience? We have heard that you, the ruler of your honorable Kingdom, have an expanded heart, and you must therefore be unwilling to do to others what you would not desire to have done to yourself".

As their impassive faces testify, the Chinese are imperturbable of temper, and therefore not easily moved to anger, and though their slow-moving government has not yet followed the example set some one or two centuries ago by those of Europe in abolishing judicial torture, they cannot be called a cruel people; on the contrary, the testimony of Friar Carpini, given six hundred years ago, that they were a "kindly folk", is abundantly confirmed by those who go among them now. And kindliness and evenness of temper certainly must dispose a people to peace. That China has been able to so far keep the peace within her borders as to have enabled a population of four hundred millions to come into being and subsist there, is good proof that her people are like the Eskimos, though in a less degree, it is true, averse to war, especially when it is considered that for centuries her borders have been infested with the terribly warlike Tartars, able to ravage Europe at will, yet whom she generally managed to keep at bay, often invading and conquering them, annexing their territory and civilizing and assimilating its inhabitants; as she did, too, when herself conquered, with the hordes that poured in under Jenghis Khan and his descendants and also with the Manchus, when, upon the invitation of one party in a civil war, they slipped in and gained possession of the government, Chinese rulers have habitually sought to avoid war by diplomacy and concessions, and by delays which give the blood time to cool. The great wall is a monument to their love of peace, and they have even made terms with pirates and given important offices to their chiefs. Chinese sages in their teachings insist upon peace as a condition essential to the well-being of the people. Lao-Tsee says of the wise ruler that "if he triumphs (in war) he does not rejoice. To rejoice is to love to kill men. He who loves to kill men cannot succeed in governing the Empire". And again : " He who has killed a multitude of men must weep over them with tears and sobs. He who has been victorious in battle they place according to the funeral rites". This last is explained in a note thus: " In antiquity, when a general had gained a victory, he put on mourning. He put himself (in the temple) in the place of those who preside at funeral rites, and, clothed in close vestments, he wept and sobbed". Twenty-five hundred years ago this denunciation of war was uttered, and the custom alluded to as prevailing in what had then become antiquity may have been still older by another like term of time. The aversion to war shown by the foregoing has doubtless grown weaker with the lapse of time. The necessity of repelling invasion by neighboring peoples of ferocious dispositions, and of sometimes absorbing them must needs in some degree have assimilated the Chinese heart to that of the Christian West, which is quite too patriotic to mourn for dead enemies, but prefers to celebrate victories by hymns of thanks and praise loud and fervent in proportion to the numbers of them killed, wounded and missing. But the fact that twenty-five hundred, perhaps five thousand years ago, it was not so is the more worthy to be noted in this connection, for the further back into the past the existence of such peaceable dispositions can be traced the more creditable it is to the original stock whence the Chinese have descended, and the more close the resemblance grows between them and the Eskimos, and the likelihood that that stock was the root race of both.

Another point of resemblance in the customs of the two people is found in their treatment of persons moribund. On an earlier page the Eskimo custom in this respect has been described; that of the Chinese is singularly like it. An account of the "dead house" in the Chinese quarter of San Francisco says: "The dying receive little or no attention and are generally hustled off to the death houses, where they end their days amid such grim surroundings as the boxed-up bones of Chinamen awaiting shipment home. Often they die unattended".

Let us imagine a portion of the cave-dwellers on their tramp northward to have detached themselves from the rest, and by force of circumstances easily imagined, become warlike enough to go where they pleased in search of a desirable habitat. They would naturally turn their steps southward, and as they got into warmer regions than those where the temperature of their dwellings of snow had to be kept below freezing point, lest they should melt away, where clothes of fur were necessary even in summer time, and where scarcity of fuel forced them to eat their food uncooked, they would soon discard their clothing, and, of course, have no need of fire. Now, Chinese history begins with describing the nucleus of the Chinese Nation as "a little horde of wanderers roving among the forests of Shan-se, without houses, without clothing, without fire to dress their victuals, and subsisting on the spoils of the chase, eked out with roots and insects", who, coming from down the North, established small colonies on the fertile plains of the modern province of that name, and, settling there, ceased to be nomads and became agriculturalists. There, history goes on to say, they were able to repel invasion from the aborigines, for which purpose only defensive ferocity was necessary, and in aid of which, as a means of securing peace, we may readily suppose they brought to bear the same spirit of fair dealing which now prompts the Greenlanders in their commerce with the Danes to leave it for the latter to fix the price of what they purchase, and which prompted Penn, the Quaker, in his dealings with the red men of Pennsylvania, to act justly so that of the treaty he made with them Voltaire could say that it was the only one never sworn to, and the only one never broken. And thus enjoying peace and plenty, only such qualities of mind and heart as those Greenlanders now so notably evince were needed to ensure for the new nation, while yet its blood was uncontaminated with Tartar mixtures, the attainment of a civilization worthily named " hospitable and contemplative", rendering the enjoyers of it "mild, just and frugal, kindly and polished". If the development thus favorably begun and for a long period rapidly progressing has been arrested, as it is often remarked that Chinese civilization seems to have been, it should be charged to the account of war and the Tartars. The oblique eyes of the Chinese, which is considered good proof that they came originally from the far North, again assimilates them to the Eskimos. But do they not still remain as oval-eyed as these last ? If they do the question arises: If six or eight thousand years have not sufficed to efface the supposed effects of the snow-glare in any clearly perceptible degree, how many years of exposure to snow-glare was needed to so impress its stamp in the first place ? A question relating to the antiquity of man. That the Eskimos are as good as a people need be, and at the same time singularly adverse to warfare, will by most men be accepted as proving not only that peaceful conditions favor the evolution of goodness, but that they are essential to it. Unfortunately it proves also that a people who will not fight cannot hold their own in this warring world, so as to exemplify on any large scale the advantages of goodness. Driven out of the habitable world, the cave-dwellers and their descendants have had small chance for converting their goodness into happiness, and soon their seed will be known no more on land or snow, and their pattern lost forever. Certainly, the evolutionary experiment in their case of making a people good in conduct by means of security and peace has been a failure. At best a hint and a hope is all the world has got from the example of the forty thousand who yet crouch in caves or ice tomes, dirty and vermin-bitten, contented though they be. And for aught we know, many a race as good and peaceful as they may before now have been swept out of existence by races ferocious and bad as we. Yet untiring evolution still goes on as if aiming at creating some time or other a world wherein good men can live and peaceful races persist. But how? The influences which have availed to secure orderly conditions within territorial limits of nations seem never to have come into play beyond such limits. Neither the law of love nor the golden rule, both considered so good in respect to dealings of man with man, seems yet to have been thought of as applying to dealings of nation with nation. And yet if man is ever to attain to any ideal state of goodness it must be while sheltered by long-continued peaceful conditions. The problem to solve is how a peaceable nation can keep its peace without going to war. Perhaps the superior mechanical skill and greater wealth of European nations may yet become joined to peaceful dispositions and furnish the solution.

CHAPTER XVII - HINDU YOGA

According to the Vedanta philosophy man first becomes man when he forgets he is god. He is created by nothing but the obscuration of his own consciousness, and he can again become god simply by returning to his original knowledge of himself. Thus he may re-discover himself and know that he has always been god. It is this re-discovery of himself that the Sanskrit word yoga, literally joined, is commonly used to express. But the re-discovery is not made as knowledge is ordinarily obtained ; and the searcher must undergo a sort of transformation before he can receive it. It is only in the last stage to which persistent practice can consciously carry the yogi, that of Samadhi, that it comes to him as an ecstatic influx touching at once both intellect and will, filling the one with light and the other with joy, as if in tracing his lineage backward towards its beginning he had come to that link in the chain of causation where love and wisdom are as yet undivergent, and can be conceived only as one. The means or ways of attaining yoga, which we will term "yoga practice", all resolve themselves into concentration of mind. And to this concentration Hinduism, which is both philosophy and religion, makes all its vast collection of gods of every degree, all its countless temples, with their idols and symbols, in which those gods are worshipped, all its theology and ritual of devotion, but the subservient means. For yoga is above and beyond all these; they merely conduct the devotee up to it, and at its portals vanish as guides and ushers should. To the whole thing, the work and what is worked for, the term yoga is commonly applied, just as in old Chinese literature the word tao is, which can mean way to travel on, but when used in relation to the practice in question means the way in which it is performed, the method, art and mystery of it, as plainly appears on pages 233, 239 and 251 of Mr. Giles' translation of Chaung Tzü wherein it is also sometimes made to mean the first principle of Nature, or the one impersonal God. But the same Chinese word, when placed as second syllable in "Shinto", which means literally "way of the gods", seems there to signify a way to travel on, leading to a paradise called "The Land of the Gods", and not to a state of being, which Hindu Yoga may be properly termed.

Vedantism does not recognize yoga practice as good for any other purpose than getting out of earth-life and getting back to Brahman, and thereby obtaining release from repeated re-births which must otherwise go on in a series without end while the present universe lasts. Accordingly, the supernatural gifts that come of it are disregarded as disturbing allurements merely, not worth being considered by one who treads the path that leads to the god, that himself is. Müller has truly said that we know very little about yoga. Possibly he thinks it beneath an European's notice. Others, willing to notice it, have ventured the guess that all its incontestable phenomena are due to self-magnetism, but the persevering student for whose benefit the following summary of the principal systems of yoga of which we have accounts have been made, will be more likely to dismiss the self-magnetism theory as far too scant to cover the facts, and to find in them the stirring of an inner man quite worthy to be named soul, attended by phenomena which go towards proving experimentally, and not inspirationally, emotionally or metaphysically, that man in his wholeness is a being great enough to be trusted with his own destiny. If a study of yoga should result in the conclusion that its whole meaning has never yet been found out; it would not be wonderful, for the world is yet young. And the true student should not be sorry to know that a field of investigation had opened before him of wider extent than any other that has yet been explored, or even known to exist.

Hatha Yoga

Quietude being essential to yoga it could not have arisen in very early and therefore rude and turbulent times, as there is proof that ancestor worship did. But it is old enough to be largely treated of in the primitive Hindu scripture. The Vedas contain it, the Upanishads, for instance, being devoted principally to it, and the Vedanta gives name to what is considered its higher branch. The other or lower branch, however, must have come first, because it is the more simple and practical and the less religious and philosophical, and because its phenomena will be seen to have furnished the basis on which Hindu metaphysics was built, or at least to have furnished hints for the hypotheses which formed that basis. Therefore the Hatha has precedence here of the Vedanta or Rajah.

An approved presentation of the former is "the Hatha Yoga Pradipika " of Swatmaram Swami, of which an English translation was published in 1893. Of its four chapters the first contains some introductory matter — a caution to secrecy, a description of a proper habitation for the student or practicer, which must be secluded but pleasant and with agreeable surroundings — prescribes correct habits and good moral conduct and certain religious observances — directs the postures proper to be assumed in performing the various exercises, which postures, however, may be here omitted as unsuited to people who do not sit cross-legged, though much stress is laid upon them in the book, which enjoins, in connection with them, certain mental attitude, such as contemplating on Brahman, concentrating on the Nadis or sounds coming from the yogin's own breast, and fixing the eyes on the tip of the nose with a concentrated mind. The chapter also recommends a moderate diet, defined to mean pleasant and sweet food in quantity to leave one-fourth of the stomach empty. The second chapter treats pranyama, or breathing practice. It prescribes various methods for drawing in, retaining and letting out the breath, for exhaling and holding out, and for arresting the breathing without regard to inhalation or exhalation. Furaka is the term for inhalation, Rechaka the one for exhalation, and Kumbhaka the one for retention. Here is an example of these methods. " The yogi, assuming the Padmasana posture (each breathing has its appropriate posture) should draw in the Prana (breath) through the Ida, or left nostril, and having retained it as long as he can, exhale it through the Pingala or right nostril. Again inhaling the Prana through the Pingala, he should per form Kumbhaka (retention) as laid down in the books, and should again slowly exhale it through the Ida. He should perform Puraka (inhalation) through the same nostril by which he performed Rechaka, and having restrained the breath to the utmost (till he is covered with perspiration or till his body shakes), should exhale it slowly and never fast, as that would diminish the energy of the body". He should perform these breathings four times a day — in the early morning, at mid-day, evening and midnight, slowly increasing the number from three each time to eighty. The effect is to "render the body slender and bright". Although in the translation the Ida is named as being the left nostril and the Pingala as the right one, these words more appropriately designate two supposed conduits which connect with the nostrils and thence conduct throughout the whole body a certain vital air that enters with the atmosphere air, but is quite a different thing from it. The Ida is said to lie on the left and the Pingala on the right of another more important conduit named the Sushumna. All three are again included in the term nadi, of which there are supposed to be seventy-two thousand, all leading down from the throat to the Kundali, in the pelvic region, and connecting with it.

Yogis of phlegmatic temperament are directed to go through a course of preparation before undertaking Pranayama, which course consists in: (1) cleansing the gullet with a strip of cloth swallowed and then withdrawn (the first introduction to be gradual, at the rate of one span's length daily); (2) enemas of water; (3) cleansing the nostrils by putting up a thread and drawing it out by way of the mouth; (4) looking without winking at a minute object with concentrated mind till tears come; (5) with head bent down turning the viscera of the body to right and left; (6) breathing in and out rapidly, like a blacksmith's bellows. Internal concentration causing the stomach to empty itself by vomiting is also recommended.

When by a proper course of Pranayama the nadis have been purified, the breath easily forces itself into the mouth of the Sushumna and enters it. This gives "steadiness to the mind", and various miraculous powers result. The signs of perfection in Hatha Yoga are: "the body becomes lean, the speech eloquent, the inner sounds (to be hereafter mentioned in detail) are distinctly heard, the eyes are clear and bright, the body is freed from all disease, the seminal fluid is concentrated, the digestive fire is increased and the nadis are purified".

Next there is a description of three Bandhas: "The Uddiana Bandha" says the commentary, "seem to be this : By a very strong expiration the lungs are emptied and driven against the upper part of the thorax, carrying the diaphragm along with them, and the intestines are taken up and fill the vacant space". The stomach is by this made so slender it might be compassed by a span. Mula Bandha is this: Pressing the Yoni with the ankle, contract the anus and draw upwards the Apana (or downward flowing breath). Again, " Pressing the anus with the ankle, contract the air forcibly and constantly until the breath goes upwards".

To perform the Jalandhara Bandha "contract the throat and press the chin firmly against the breast (four inches from the heart)". The Viparitakarani Bandha, which is practiced for the purpose of making the " moon", which is at the root of the palate, change places with the "sun", which is near the navel, is to be learned only from the teacher.

The third chapter treats of the ten Mudras which are to be practiced for the purpose of "rousing the great goddess Kundalini who sleeps closing the (lower) mouth of the Sushumna". These are said to "destroy old age and death", having been given out by the god Siva, and to confer the eight Siddhis, or miraculous powers. They are much sought after by all Siddhas (possessors of such powers) and are difficult to obtain even by the Devas (lesser gods). Concerning them it is added: "This should be carefully kept secret as a box of diamonds and should not be told to anybody — just as the illicit connection with a married woman of noble family".

Maha Mudra, the first of the ten, is thus performed : " Pressing the anus with the left heel and stretching out the right leg, take hold of the toes with your hand. Then practice the Jalandhara Bandha (lately described), and draw the breath through the Sushumna. Then the Kundalini becomes straight, just as a coiled snake does when struck, and the Ida and Pingala become dead, because the breath goes out of them. Then the breath should be let out very slowly, and never quickly". Maha Bandha (sic.) comes next, and is thus described: "Having restrained the breath as long as possible he should then breathe out slowly. He should practice first on the left side and then on the right". This is said to stop the upward course of the breath through the Nadis except Sushumna, and bring about the union of them with the Sushumna, and also to " enable the mind to remain fixed between the two eyebrows".

But these two Mudras are said to have no value without a third named the Maha Vedha, which is to be thus performed: The yogi . . . " should draw in his breath with a concentrated mind and stop the upward and downward course of the breath by the Jalandhara Bandha. Resting at the same time his body on his hands placed on the ground, he should repeatedly but gently seat and raise himself. The body assumes a deathlike aspect. Then he should breathe out". The Kechari Mudra requires the following preparation : By slight daily repeated cuttings continued during six months, the ligament is severed that holds down the tongue, which then, by repeatedly pulling it out, is made long enough to touch the eyebrows. The Mudra is performed by turning up the tongue and making it enter the hole in the palate where the three Nadis join, at the same time "fixing the eyes firmly between the brows".

The Vajroli Mudra which is said to give the five Siddhis even to one who lives an ordinary life, with the Amaroli and Sahajoli which are kindred to it, occupy twenty Sutras which remain untranslated on account of their peculiar character, and will not be further noticed here for the reasons that the commentary claims that they are not to be understood literally and are besides incomplete in some points, which are left to be filled by verbal instructions of the guru. If any such arcanum as this Vajroli lie in yoga it will be apt to disclose itself soon or late to the practicer who perseveres.

The Shakati Chalana, named as the last of the ten mudras, is next described. Having inhaled through the right nostril the yogin should retain the breath in a peculiar way to be learned only from a Guru, and "manipulate the Kundalini for about an hour and a half, both at morning and evening twilights. "Some light might be obtained regarding what is thus left obscure by referring to the context, of which here are a few passages: "As one forces open a door with a key, so should the yogi force open the door of Moksha (state of bliss) by the Kundalini". "The Kundalini gives Mukti (deliverance) to the Yogis and bondage to the fools. He who knows her knows Yoga". "He who causes that Shakti (the Kundalini) to move (from the Muladhara in the pelvic region upwards) is freed without doubt". " Between the Ganges (Ida) and Jamuna (Pingala) there sits the young widow inspiring pity. He (the Yogi) should despoil her forcibly, for it leads one to the supreme seat of Vishnu". " You should awake the sleeping serpent (Kundalini) by taking hold of its tail". "Seated in the Vajrasena posture, firmly take hold of the feet near the ankle and slowly beat with them "Kanda" (a something below the navel from which the 72,000 Nadis issue). "By moving the Kundalini fearlessly for about an hour and a half, she is drawn upwards a little through the Sushumna", which process it is said " surely opens the mouth of the Sushumna and the breath naturally goes through it". Whether by manipulation of the Kundalini or other means this effect is produced, it seems to be the object primarily aimed at in Hatha Yoga work. The fruits of the practice of Hatha Yoga, taken in the order of their mention, are the following:

1. The eight Siddhis, viz. : anima (the power to assimilate oneself with an atom) ; mahima (the power to expand oneself into space) ; taghima (the power to be as light as cotton or other similar thing) ; garima (the power to grow as heavy as anything) ; prapti (the power of reaching anywhere, even to the moon) ; prakamya (the power of having all wishes of whatever description realized); isatva (power to create) ; vasitva (power to command all). 2. Freedom from death and from old age. 3. Rejuvenescence and perpetual youth. 4. Beauty. 5. Ability to "do and undo". 6. Exemption from hunger and thirst, also from indo lence. 7. Floating on water. 8. The attainment of anything in the three worlds. 9. Invulnerability to poisons. 10. Removal of wrinkles and gray hair. 11. Freedom from disease. 12. Exemption from the effects of Karma. 13. Immortality and the eight Siddhis (named above). 14. Power to attract the damsels of the Siddhas (or Mahatmas). Finally, and far beyond the Siddhis, comes the grand result of Mukti or emancipation (from re-birth) and conscious junction with Brahman.

These powers are certainly all could be desired; in fact they stop nowhere short of omnipotence, omnipresence and omniscience. But we must allow for Eastern hyperbole.

According to the commentary the fourth and last chapter is wholly devoted to Rajah Yoga. But a careful study of the book will probably convince the reader that it cannot thus be divided in two parts unless by a wrenching that does violence to its meaning as a whole; and show, moreover, that as a whole the proper title of it is Hatha Yoga. This fourth chapter may be a sort of supplement that in course of time has grown upon the original compilation. It deals a good deal with the results of the methods of practice contained in the others, specifying Rajah Yoga as one of them, and it amplifies some of those methods, but gives no new ones.

American Experiences

It is in common experience that long and close concentration upon any given part of the body will induce in it sensations, and sometimes even movements. Control over unused muscles may in that way be obtained. An experienced physician will tell his patient to keep his mind off his carbuncle, and "Don't think about your disease" is every-day advice given by visiting neighbors. While it is claimed for Hatha Yoga that the breathings can exert control over the mind through their function of supplying arterialized blood to the brain, thus controlling mental by physical action, it is on the other hand claimed that mere persistent concentration of the mind will set up those very breathings, thus controlling physical action by mental. And a story is related of a student whose teacher made him sit meditating in silence twelve years, and at last commanded him to pronounce the sacred word O. M. (which is often divided into three syllables, thus AUM). He did so, with the following result:

"When the Sanyasi came to the first syllable, Rechaka, or the process by which the air in the lungs is pumped out, set in naturally. When he finished the second syllable, Puraka, or the process of inhalation, set in. At the end of the third syllable, Kumbhaka, or the process of retention, set in". And then all else immediately followed. "In a short time he had passed the initial stages of Pratyshara, Dhyana and Dharana, and settled into the pure and elevated state of Samadhi".

This story, whether true or not, illustrates the largeness of the claim in behalf of mental yoga that it brings physical yoga with it, provided the mental processes take the form of long-continued silent concentration, and also the further claim that what it thus brings is important, since the Pranyama of the student brought him soon into perfect absorption. But both points are better illustrated by phenomena, which, if not known in India, have been experienced here in America and in these times, as will presently be shown in detail. And the occurrence of these modern phenomena also suggests the thought that like occurrences in remote times may have given rise to the postures, breathings and movements which make up the Hatha practice, whose origin, so bizarre and anomalous are they, might else remain unaccounted for. Some contemplative solitary in the valley of the Indus may, as a consequence of long concentrating on a star, an idea, or on vacancy, have found himself moved to perform involuntarily all the Kumbhakas and Mudras in their various combinations; and these being found to be associated with magical power others may have, with volition, imitated them in hopes to obtain like power. Thus Hatha Yoga may have originated. What has of late years come to my knowledge as occurring in this country after long practice of simple concentration, undertaken without any thought of yoga or knowledge that there was such a thing, is the following:

To begin with the Asanas. These, though unsuited to people who sit in chairs, have nevertheless persistently tried to force themselves upon the practicers. A leg has jerked itself upward and pressed the sole of its foot against the other as high up as seemed possible ; this has happened hundreds of times. The posture here imitated is sitting on a foot, and its efficacy is supposed to lie in the pressure upon nerve-centres in the foot, leg and region of the perineum. Another asana resembling the "plant balance" of modern gymnastics is described thus: "Plant your hands firmly on the ground and support your body on your elbows, pressing against the sides of your loins. Raise your feet in the air stiff and straight on a level with the head". This position was distinctly attempted while the practicer was seated in an easy chair, and only failed of completeness because the back of it kept the head from falling to the level of the feet. The legs were lifted from the floor and thrust out stiffly, while the weight of the whole body, except the head, was made to rest on the elbows, they resting on the arms of the chair. The attempt was repeated only once, but a great number of times the elbows were pressed against the sides with a force that seemingly could not have been voluntarily exerted, and as often have hammered themselves violently and repeatedly against the sides,giving excellent massage to both liver and spleen — though this could hardly be called an asana. The Shavasana "for removing fatigue and inducing calmness of mind " is described as lying on one's back at full length, like a corpse. Often when lying on his side the practicer has been turned over on his back, not impelled to turn by any influence acting upon his will, but turned as by a power foreign to it, though apparently using his own muscles. A curious sensation often felt seemed intended to reproduce on the feet, ankles, and seat of the body, the compression which is obtainable by sitting on the feet, Eastern fashion. It was just as if a foreign body were pressed against the parts with a force equal to what they would feel in the positions of Hatha Yoga. Sometimes several of the parts in question were thus simultaneously acted on.

The Mudras. Of these, one termed The Maha Vedha, is performed by slightly rising and reseating one's self gently and repeatedly. This was exactly reproduced. One of the six acts recommended for putting in good bodily condition those who would practice yoga is the Nauli, thus described: "With the head bent down one should turn right and left the intestines of the stomach with the slow motion of a small eddy in the river", Something like this interior movement is produced by one process of the Swedish movement-cure. It consists in sitting on a stool, bending forward as far as possible, and making the trunk of the body to rotate like the spoke of a horizontal wheel, the head representing the tire and the seat the hub. Now, it was just this Swedish movement that, in the case of two persons, was set up as often as Kumbhaka was practiced; neither of them having an idea of such a result. The nauli mudra is stated to be the most important of all the Hatha practices, and the bodily rotation is certainly one of the most effective of the Swedish ones.

"Looking fixedly at the spot between the eyebrows" is in several places named and enjoined. This was reproduced numberless times, extending through many years. Thinking of nothing seemed most readily to have that effect. The eyeballs would as of themselves roll upward as far as they could go, and hold themselves there.

The Shambhavi-mudra consists in fixing the mind on some part of the body, and the eyes rigidly and unwinking on some external object. Many times while the practicer was concentrating intently, with his eyes closed, they would open of themselves and fix on some object within their range, always rigidly and without winking, or any impulse to do so, while the concentration, whatever may have been the objective of it, went on as before.

"Direct the pupils of the eyes towards the light by raising the eyebrows a little upwards", says the book. Often the eyebrows raised themselves as if to get out of the way of the eyes. In all the above, as well as in the movements next to be described, an intelligent power beyond reach of the consciousness of the practicer seemed, so to speak, to take him out of his own hands, to assume control of his voluntary as well as involuntary muscles and work them independently of his will, though, it should be noted, never against it.

The Bandhas are movements of the internal organs by means of voluntary muscles, outside of and near them. One of these, for instance, requires that certain muscular contractions be made which will have the effect of forcing the breath to flow through the Sushumna, "being drawn in through the back part of the navel". This seems ridiculous enough, but the fact that such muscular contractions and many others have spontaneously resulted from mental concentration, no matter on what, though it cannot make sense of the Hindu three-thousand-year-old theory of anatomy, may make credible the facts it undertakes to interpret. The movements here alluded to were frequent, sudden and violent, extending now throughout the whole trunk, giving each of its organs a salutary "massage", and now involving the legs and arms. One thus handled could not but be reminded by it of the Swedish movement-cure, if he had ever tried it, though the yoga exercises far excelled in force as well as in variety those of the cure. Sometimes the muscles of the front of the chest and abdomen would jerk themselves together violently, making a cable of themselves that reached from pelvis to throat, and sometimes the same movement would be directed downward, pushing everything as far as it would go. Again the whole contents of the abdomen would be drawn up and against the backbone, and then pushed forward so as to swell them out tensely. Again the abdomen and chest would, by turns, be, the one swelled out and the other simultaneously shrunk in, and this, though repeatedly done, without noticeable movement of the breath. Again the muscles about the navel would, as it were, draw together in a knot all the organs of the region, squeezing them violently while the flanks shrunk as violently in. In short, every conceivable combination of movement by which the muscles of the trunk can act upon the contents of it, were at times gone through, and all, be it noted, in a progressive way, step by step, and each step, once attained, held on to. It is furthermore noteworthy that when a given movement, of the sort which has just been described, or one of the breathings yet to be described, had been led up to by a series of progressive ones culminating in it only after weeks or months of practice, then each subsequent repetition of it would usually be achieved in the same progressive way, seemingly as if, for a time at least, the more difficult had to be preceded by a practice of the less difficult in serial order, as well after the point of perfection had been reached as before, each repetition being a brief rehearsal of the long course of practice by which expertness in it had been acquired. The movements just described reproduce all of the important exercises called mudras, whose office is to rouse up the great goddess (Kundalini), except the Vajroli, and its modifications the Sahajoli and Amaroli, which requires two practicers, the Viparitakarani, the method of which is not disclosed, but left for the teacher to impart, and the Kechari, which requires the ligament holding down the tongue to be first cut; though a rolling backward of the tongue against the palate has been repeatedly attempted, and carried as far as could be without that mutilation; the excepted ones being by their nature not reproducible by a single person untaught by an Indian Guru, and with an uncut tongue. The distinctive marks by which these recent results of mental concentration can be identified with Hatha Yoga are such as leave no room for supposing mere coincidence of mistake.

The Uddiana Bandha that has been before described was reproduced in a manner that in every detail was perfect, and the rapidity with which the lungs would fly upward, expelling thereby all air in them, was startling.

The eight Kumbhakas, or breathings, named in the book, were reproduced with equal fidelity except in the following respects: The nostrils were not closed with the fingers, nor the tongue placed between or protruded through the lips, nor any hissing sounds made in drawing in or letting out the breath, though the tongue made efforts to push itself forward, and distinctly, as just said, rolled itself back against the palate as if attempting the Kechari Mudra. The breath seemed to draw itself in, hold itself there and let itself out, and the head would bend downward so as to press the chin against the breast, as directed in the manual, for the purpose of making the retention easy. And when thus retained the air seemed to expand so that the practicer would feel it "pervade the whole of his body from the head to the toe", as the book expresses it. There was no distinction made as to which nostril the breath should enter or depart by, as in the book, but the inhaling, retaining and exhaling, the expelling, excluding and inhaling, and the simple stop-page in mid-breathing and "holding the breath", all came as the book directs, and without conscious volition.

As a result, or at least an incident of our American experiments, there came a remarkable series of self-manipulations which might be likened to mesmeric passes or massage movements. The mind of the operator not consciously concurring, they could hardly be classed with the one, and not being known to any system of massage could hardly belong with the other, but they resembled both. Like the reproductions of the Mudras and Kumbhakas, they arose quite independently of, though never against, the will of the practicer. It would be safe to say there were a hundred of them, of all degrees of emphasis, from the gentle tapping of a finger to the violent kicking out of a leg; all following at the touch of a mere thought, as it were — no, of a mental effort in arrest of thought — and as quickly as any electric effect follows the touching of a button. Though the manipulations were mostly made with abnormal force and without consciousness of any effort but the mental one, and generally left a sense of well being, it would be inexact to say there was no resulting fatigue, yet there was certainly less that must have followed intentional exercises of a like sort. There were no unmeaning movements, but all seemed to be devised with masterly skill, aiming at curative effects, while to the practicer each one of them was new and original, and on its first occurrence a surprise.

Sankhya Yoga.

Quite unlike the hand-book of yoga practice, which Swatmaram's work may be termed, are the Sutras of the Sage Kapila believed to be no other than god Vishnou, son of Brahman, in the fifth of his twenty-four incarnations. These seem to be merely a series of philosophical propositions, yet their propounder claims that the study of them will surely conduct to Samadhi and deliverance. Though the Sankhya philosophy admits that the ills of life may be palliated and a temporary release from re-births be obtained, by temporal means discoverable by reason, and devotional observances revealed by God, yet it declares that complete and final deliverance from re-birth can only be attained by what is termed: "A method different from both, consisting in a discriminative knowledge of perceptible principles, and of the imperceptible one, and of the thinking soul " — or, as more fully set forth by the commentary: " The accurate discrimination of those principles into which all that exists is distributed by the Sankhya philosophy; Vyakta, that which is perceived, sensible, discreet; Avyakta, that which is unperceived, indiscreet, and Jna, that which knows, or discriminates. The first is matter in its perceptible modifications; the second is crude, unmodified matter, and the third is soul. The object of the Sankhya Yoga is to define and explain these three things, the correct knowledge of which is in itself release from worldly bondage and exemption from exposure to human ills, by the final separation of soul and body".

There is nothing said by this sage of any postures, movements or breathings of the body, or of any effort of the mind save what is implied in any philosophical study. In other yogas the knowledge that sets the soul free from re-birth is supposed to come at the end of a long course of practice of one kind or other, and in form of intuition or spiritual impression such as makes the saint to know the truth after he has quite lost his reason in ecstatic entrancement. But Kapilas' teaching seems to be addressed to the waking reason alone, unenlightened by any supernatural influx.

Yet following on the promulgation of this Sankhya philosophy (so called from its being an enumeration or analysis of the universe), and claiming to be in general accordance with it, came an elaborate system of Sankhya Yoga, first embodied in the Sutras of Patanjali, a work written as early as the seventh century A. D., and of high authority, A sample of his method of intellectualizing magic practice is found in the following verses:

" 1. Now an exposition of yoga is to be made".

" 2. Yoga is the suppression of the transformations of the thinking principle".

" 3. Then the seer abides in himself".

" 4. But otherwise becomes assimilated with transformations".

" 5. The transformations are five-fold, and are painful or not painful".

" 6. Right knowledge, wrong knowledge, fancy, sleep and memory".

" 7. Right knowledge is direct cognition, or inference, or testimony".

" 8. Wrong knowledge is a false conception of a thing whose real form does not answer to it in reality".

" 9. Fancy is the notion called into being having nothing to answer to it in reality".

"10. That transformation which has nothingness for its basis is sleep".

" II. Memory is not allowing a thing cognized to escape".

"12. Its suppression is secured by application and non-attachment".

" 13. Application is the effort towards the state (Stilhi) in which the mind is at a stand-still".

" 14. It becomes a position of firmness being practiced for a long time without intermission and with perfect devotion".

" 15. The consciousness of having mastered (every desire) in the case of one who does not thirst for objects perceptible or scriptural, is nonattachment".

" 16. That is highest wherein, from being the Purusa (soul) there is entire cessation of any, the least desire for the Gunas (things of sense)".

The yoga practice recommended by Patanjali consists in meditation on Kapilas' 25 categories or Tattvas, — the exercise of faith, energy, memory and discriminative judgment, ardent desire to attain to Samadhi, devotion to Iswara a god invented to help contemplation, constant repetition of and intent meditation on his "word of glory", O M, intense concentration on some one thing, sympathy with happiness, compassion for misery, complacency towards virtue and indifference to evil, the breathings (Pranyama), concentration on any sensuous enjoyment by those who cannot steady their minds but through some kind of sensual pleasure, which is done, according to the commentary, by "fixing the attention on one of the five senses of smell, taste, color, touch and sound. These are respectively produced by concentrating on the tip of the nose, the tip of the tongue, the forepart of the palate, the middle of the tongue, and the root of the tongue. The sensation produced in each case is not merely a passing flash of pleasurable feeling; but a kind of complete absorption in the particular enjoyment meditated upon". Then there is concentration on the Joytis (light), and to help concentration it is to be imagined that in the heart there is a lotus-like form having eight petals and with its face turned downward, which can be raised up by exhaling the breath, and should then be meditated on while pronouncing O M, the effect of which is that a calm light is seen "like that of the moon or sun, resembling the calm ocean of milk". Or the concentration maybe on the condition of deep sleep — or, finally, "according to one's predilection", that is to say, on any one thing.

So much for the objects of concentration. The states induced by it and other results next follow: The test of proper concentration having been acquired is "a mastery extending from the finest atom to infinity. " The two kinds of or stages in concentration, the argumentative, or mixed, and the non-argumentative, or pure, are described, and their result indicated, bliss, intuition, revelation, etc. These two stages seem to correspond to the meditation and contemplation of Christian ascetics, as will be seen later.

Preliminary Yoga is next considered, which consists of "mortification, study and resignation to Iswara", and is meant for those who have not been able to accomplish Samadhi by the methods just pointed out. Ignorance, the Sense of being, Desire, Aversion and Attachment, are named as distractions to be avoided, the nature of each is explained, and the way to overcome each by appropriate meditation is given. Accessories to this are forbearance, observance, posture, regulation of breath, abstraction, contemplation, absorption and trance, and the needed explanation is given of what these mean in respect to yoga. Thus, forbearance means abstinence from killing, falsehood, theft, incontinence and greediness; observance means purity, contentment, mortification, study and resignation to Iswara; "posture is that which is easy and steady"; regulation of the breath means the same as in Hatha Yoga; abstraction means drawing away the senses from their objects in the same way that thoughts are drawn away, abstracted, from theirs, whence "follows the greatest mastery over the senses " ; contemplation means "the fixing of the mind on something"; absorption means so fixing it that the mind and that something become one; trance is when this fixing of the mind is carried so far that the thinker, the thinking and the thing thought of are one. These last three together constitute Samyama", which is the way to several occult powers and also conducts to conscious Samadhi, the yoga proper, while the five other accessories are called external means, being useful only in obviating distractions. But even this falls short of real or unconscious Samadhi, the final end of yoga, which is, says Patanjati, " that condition of the mind which is transformation into unity".

Here follows a list of the Siddhis, or miraculous powers, with the several modes of exercising them through the performance of Samyama. They are:

1. Knowing the past and future. 2. Recollecting previous incarnations. 3. Discerning the state of a person's mind by outward signs, like complexion, tone of voice, etc. 4. Reading the thoughts of another. 5. The power to become invisible. 6. Knowing the time of one's death, by meditating on his Karma, or by portents, such as spectres, dreams, etc. 7. Attracting the good will of others. 8. Acquiring the powers of any animal, as the strength of an elephant, by meditating on it. 9. Knowing "the subtle, the obscure and the remote", by contemplating on the inner light, such as yogis are able to evoke by performing Rechaka. 10. The knowledge of space by contemplating on the sun. 11. Knowledge of the starry regions by contemplating on the moon. 12. Knowledge of the motions of the stars by contemplating on the polestar. 13. Knowledge of the internal arrangement of the body by contemplating on the important nerve-centre near the navel. The nerve-centres are termed circles, padmas, chakras, and contemplation on them is an important branch of yoga work, as set forth by Patanjali, as well as in the work on Hatha Yoga lately considered. 14. Destroying hunger and thirst by contemplating on the pit of the throat. 15. Making the body fixed and immovable by contemplating on the Kurma-nadi, a certain nerve where the vital air is supposed to reside. 16. The power of seeing the beings called Siddhas, otherwise Mahatmas, by contemplating on the light in the head, which is made to appear somewhere near the pineal gland or coronal artery, or over the medulla oblongata, by concentration on the space between the eyebrows.

17. The power to accomplish all the before named things by pratibha which is: that degree of intellect which develops itself without any special cause, generally termed "intuition", and can be developed by simply contemplating on the intellect. 18. Knowledge of the mind of another or of one's own, by contemplating on the nerve-centre of the heart. 19. Knowledge on one's soul as distinct from his mind, by contemplating on himself. 20. As resulting from this knowledge intuitional perception of all the objects of the senses, no matter how far distant in time or space. (All the foregoing siddhis are here expressly denounced both in text and commentary as obstacles in the way. Not so these which follow.)

21. Entering into and possessing another body, whether living or dead, by discovering through contemplation on the nerves the particular one by which mind can pass in and out. 22. Levitation of the body and also the ability to die at will. 23. Effulgence of the body, halos about the head, etc. Also Clairaudience, or power to hear distant sounds, by concentration on

Akâsa, the either conveying sound. 24. Ability to pass bodily through space, by concentration on the relation between the body and akâsa, as also by being identified with light substances such as cotton. 25. The condition of Mahavideha, in which "knowledge of every description is within easy reach of the ascetic", and obtainable without effort. 26. Mastery over the elements by concentrating on their natures respectively. 27. The attainment of anima and the others, as also perfection of the body and the corresponding non-obstruction of its functions. " Anima and the others " are the same " eight Siddhis " before mentioned in what related to Hatha Yoga. 28. Beauty, gracefulness and strength, adamantine hardness of body. 29. Mastery over the organs of sense by concentration on their natures. 30. As a result of this mastery, fleetness of body equal to that of mind, sensation independently of the body or its organs of sense. Ability to command any thing and create any thing at will. 31. Mastery over all things and knowledge of all, by contemplating on the "distinctive relation of soul and mind". 32. Kaivalya, the highest end, the state of oneness, of being one and alone, obtained by renouncing attachment to even these ten last-named high occult powers. It may very well be conceived that the intense thought needed to produce such a system as that of Kapila would amount to a mental concentration suficient to induce the state of mind that brings on ecstacy and lets in supernal light, just as intense and persistent devotion will; the same with the hard thinking required for understanding it by his disciples. But the truth or falsity of his propositions need have had nothing to do with either his or their yoga results. And certainly the Patanjali formulation contains enough of concentrative work to carry the practicer along on the path, though the student should lag behind. The same disposition that was shown by Kapila to rely on intellectual convictions — a reliance condemned by all the magicians of old, I think — is manifested at the present day by the many schools of magical healers, each of which claims to cure by simply telling the patient the one only truth, which it alone and none other possesses. Neither truth nor untruth can be shown to have magical power, but concentration on any lie or any truth, long kept up, will still the mind and thereby let in Nature to do her work. And if she, adapting her methods to her material, at the same time that she develops them as yogis, humors the preconceptions of those she acts on, so as to reveal to each the truth he likes best, now telling the Hindu saint that he is Brahman, and now confirming the good Catholic in his belief in Papal infallibility, her doing so leaves both propositions no truer than they were before, — and such, doubtless, was the opinion of Kapila when he set up reason against revelation; though when, by force of concentration on the construction of his system, he had attained to Samadhi in its ultimate stage where spiritual impressions flow in, and such impressions confirmed him in his previous conclusions and revealed to him that release obtained by his methods was complete and final, and all others incomplete and temporary, something he has not in his aphorisms attempted to prove in any other way, naturally he must have felt that he had both reason and revelation on his side. But reason is no more infallible than its mystical offspring revelation, and the modern yogi will be the wiser the more he practices and the less he theorizes.

The Rajah Yoga Philosophy of S'rimat Sankaracharya.

In his treatise on direct cognition of the unity of the soul with Brahman, this famous teacher begins by enjoining on the practicer indifference to all life's pleasures, patience under its pains, a fixed theoretical determination that nothing is real but the Self (Atman) — desire to obtain release, and right thinking, which last means acceptance of the author's doctrines.

After abundantly and clearly setting forth all these he comes down to practical work in verse loo, which is as follows: "Henceforward (for the instruction of those who require to be taken step by step to the realization of the said truth) we begin to propound the fifteen stages necessary for the acquisition of the knowledge described before. Knowing all these one must use all of them towards acquiring a habit of constant, firm and active meditation". These stages are : (1) Yama, or restraint over the senses; (2) Niyama, or constant consciousness of unity with Brahman ; (3) Tyaga, recognition of Brahman as being everywhere; (4) Mauna, "that indescribable Brahman" which, though the mind turns back baffled from it, the learned must ever try to possess; (5) Des'a, of which all said is, "That is the real solitary De's (place) wherein the universe does not exist in the beginning, middle or end; and which is to be found through the whole of this (material) life"; (6) Kula, or the support and sustenance of all actions and the real and only fountain of joy; (7) Asana, or position assumed when meditating or practicing physical exercises — the one found most easy being the best; (8) Mulabandha, of which all said, is: "That which is the origin of all being, and that on whom depends the original (ignorance) obstruction of the manas (sic)., is the Mulabandha, to be always practiced, and is the only one to be taken up by students of Rajah or mental Yoga (to the exclusion of the rather phalic bandhas of Hatha Yoga); (9) Dehasamya, a mental method for straightening the body, for which physical movements are sometimes practiced; (10) Drikathiti, which consists in viewing with the mind's eye the whole universe as Brahman, or knowing the seer, the sight and the thing seen as one, a mental substitute for looking at the tip of the nose. (11) Pranasamyama, or "the constant and permanent obstruction of all the senses (internal) through the process of viewing all objects such as the mind and its creations as in and of Brahman", a substitute for the breathings of Hatha, Yoga, in which such viewing stands for Rechaka (breathing out), the conviction " I am Brahman" stands for Puraka (breathing in), and concentration on that conviction stands for Kumbhaka (holding the breath in); (12) Pratyahara, or the resolving all objects into Atman; (13) Dharna, or steadying the mind by making it " recognize Brahman wherever it travels or goes"; (14) Atmadhyana, or condition of highest joy arising from the conviction, " I am Brahman"; (15) Samadhi (of the unconscious sort) or " the negation of all mental action, by the mind's being reduced to a state beyond all change, and by its being ever merged in Brahman".

This course, it is said, is to be studied only so long as is needed for the yogis to "acquire the power of, at the spur of the moment, collecting and concentrating themselves". The following are the closing verses of the treatise :

" 143. This with the parts set forth above is Rajah or mental Yoga mixed with Hatha or physical Yoga, prescribed for those who have already lost a portion of their taste for the pleasures of the senses".

" 144. To those whose minds are completely ripe this Rajah Yoga alone (without any Hatha or physical Yoga) is useful ; this yoga again being one easily accessible even to those who are devoted to their teachers, or to their favorite gods, etc."

In the Vedant Sara, composed from a comment written by Sankaracharya on the Vedanta, it is said "to point out that the knowledge of Brahman was the only certain way of obtaining liberation instead of the severe mortifications of former yogis, which mankind at present are incapable of performing, and to destroy among men attachment to works of merit", it is argued that though the old doctrine had been that both works and wisdom were required to obtain liberation, Sankaracharya had in his comment on the Bhagavat Gita by many proofs shown that works are wholly excluded, and that knowledge alone, realizing every thing as Brahman, procured liberation.

In the same author's celebrated "Crest Jewell of Wisdom" we find the same insistence on knowledge being the only way to liberation and Brahman, It is admitted that temporary liberation from re-birth may be obtained by means of good Karma and religious observances, etc., but it is asserted that permanent salvation can only come by the knowledge of oneness with Deity through right discrimination — by knowledge of one's own soul — which knowledge is only gained "by perception, by investigation, or by instruction, but not by bathing or giving of alms, or by a hundred retentions of the breath, or any amount of Karma". Again: "Liberation cannot be achieved except by the direct perception of the identity of the individual with the universal self, neither by yoga, nor by Sankya (speculative philosophy), nor by the practice of religious ceremonies, nor by mere teaching". There seems to be some inconsistency here.

"The Philosophy and Science of Vedanta and Rajah Yoga " by the Mahatma Jnana Guru Yogi Sabhapaty Swami., is a work of our own times, the author having been born in 1840. Early in life there fell upon him that religious unrest which gives its victim no respite until soon or late the continuous and intense concentration which it induces carries him a certain ways into the state of Samahadi, in which at last he finds peace and rest, a curative crisis such as Nature has often to operate, whether for the benefit of Hindu Yogis, Catholic saints or Methodist converts. In his crisis Sabhapaty had a vision of the Infinite Spirit, by whom he was directed to go to certain holy men and be initiated, much after the manner of Saint Paul and his vision. Obedient as was the saint, and filled with as divine an ecstasy, he abandoned his family at midnight, and wrapped in only a sheet went as directed. Within a short time he attained to such a degree of Samadhi, that he could sit several days together without any food and enjoying full absorption. After nine years of yoga work, during which he lived in a cave and fed on roots, he went forth by command of his teacher to make known to the world the truths he had learned, performing as he went many notable miracles. The treatise in hand is the substance of two of his lectures, and is important as showing the latest phase of yoga. It begins with declaring the object of it to be "to show the method by which the human soul is sure to gain success in holding communion with the Universal Infinite Spirit, and thereby become the very Infinite Spirit itself".

Passing over the religious, scientific and philosophical part and coming to the practical, we have the following:

"Then imagine that you throw, or draw within, the real and actual light of your two eyes internally to kundali, which will appear the acute and keen divine sight; here the Sushumna vessel joins the lingam and ascends upwards through the backbone. The sight must be thrown in such a way that the keenness of those two sights, or the imaginary knowledge, Jnana or consciousness of these two eyes, shall descend through the right and left holes of the sushumana to the lowest point of kundali. By the keenness of sight is meant that indescribable something that seems to proceed from the eyes when you steadily gaze at a distant object with half-shut eyes".

"Now imagine the mind to be a straight pole whose top is in the middle of the Brahmarandhra (the centre of the skull) and whose bottom is in the kundali. Moreover, consider the mental vision or consciousness to be lodged in the bottom of the pole".

" Now take hold of the mental vision by the keenness of the two eyes and lift it up gradually and slowly, as with tongs, to the Brahmarandhra. The time taken in this pulling up of the mental consciousness must not be less than twenty minutes".

" Now stop this imaginary mental consciousness in the Brahmarandhra for twenty minutes more. Then drop and draw it up so fast that within a second it must descend to the kundali and re-ascend to the Brahmarandhra, running straight up and down through the middle vessel of the large Sushumna which we have considered to be the mental pole". (This middle vessel is the lesser Sushumna.)

" After practicing this for a few minutes, make your mind to stand upon the pole steady and straight as if it were fixed to a firm rocky pole. There let it stand immovable and without descending again. Make it to be in dead and calm silence, void and without motion, and free from all thoughts and fickleness".

" After succeeding in making the pole of your mind (or eternal divine conscious sight) straight and steady by the foregoing process, join the conscious sight of the two eyes with the top of the mind in the Brahmarandhra. Thus it forms a triangle whose vertex is the mind, and the two keennesses that proceed from the eyes to join the former, the two sides".

" Having got success in this practice, imagine strongly that your head is removed, and of course with it eyes, ears, nose, mouth and everything pertaining to the head. Instead of it consider that the whole space is filled up by the universal (Jnanakasha) consciousness, which now becomes the holy akâsa itself".

Next the yogin is directed to make "a divine pilgrimage in the universe of his body", the lines of it leading from the top of the head, through the Sushumna, down to the Kundali, and thence upward through the same, now termed kumbak, to starting point. Along this line are located twelve certain spirits, at each of which the mind stops and addresses to it an argumentative assertion and sings with piety an appropriate mantram, the intent of all which is to produce a realizing knowledge of the nature of body and of spirit. For instance, the mind on its way down is made to pause at the centre of the tongue where the Jivatma (infinite spirit) becomes the finite spirit of consciousness, appearing in three forms, namely, as activity, darkness and goodness, and there to stand and to tell it, "I am not you", by singing with devotion some verses, and then pass on.

Finally, Pranyama, the breathings, the same as in Hatha Yoga, are prescribed, though with a protest that it is not really necessary, in which he but agrees with other teachers, who, while disparaging the older and more laborious practice, seem unable to do without it. Not only does this one include Pranyama, but the concentration he directs upon this and that part of the body is merely the Shakti process of Hatha with variations and additions.

Tatwic Yoga

"The Science of Breath " is the title of a little book translated from the Sanscrit a few years ago by the Pandit Rama Prasad, and which attracted so much notice that he afterwards embodied it in a larger volume on "Nature's Finer Force", otherwise made up of explanatory essays of his own. He says in the preface to the first that it is not a very exact translation, and the same is true of the second. Each contains matter not in the other, and there are signs that something of the original work is omitted from both, so that the reader has to piece out the one from the other in the best way he can.

As before explained, the "Breath'" treated of is not of the lungs, but "Prana", the "Great Breath", which pervades all nature, the first cause of all things, the life-giving breath of Brahman, whose out-going is creation and whose in-drawing is destruction. Of this "great breath" the five Tatwas are the first differentiation. They may be otherwise named the five states of matter, — the five elementary principles of nature, — the five modes of motion, — the five vibratory ethers. On all planes of being, spiritual, mental, psychic and physical, they correspond to the five senses of man, whose organs they create and then act upon. In Akâsa, ether par excellence, the first in order and out of which all the others are produced, which, as it were, contains them all and separates them from each other and penetrates all things, is found the sense of hearing, in Vayu (air) that of touch, in Taijas (fire) that of seeing, in Apas (water) that of taste, and in Prithivi (earth) that of smell. Each of them is produced by the one preceding it in the above stated order, and each has a vibration peculiar to itself. The tatwic philosophers assuming to have obtained knowledge of the laws of the tatwic movement through revelation as well as reason, have elaborated a philosophy covering all of nature's doing and being, the study of which as set forth by Mr. Prasad, whether its conclusions be accepted or not, is a delight to the enquiring mind. Of this philosophy the authoritative gospel is the little book in question. It says: "The universe came out of tatwa; it goes on by the instrumentality of the tatwas; it disappears in the tatwas; by the tatwas is known the nature of the universe. The knowers of the tatwas have ascertained them to be the highest root. Unmanifested, formless, the one giver of light is 'The Great Power ' ; from that appeared the soniferous ether (akâsa); from that had birth the tangiferous ether (Vayu); from the tangiferous ether, the luminiferous ether (taijas), and from this, gustiferous ether (apas); from hence was the birth of the odoriferous ether (prithivi). These are the five ethers and they have a fivefold extension. Of these the Universe came out; by these it goes on; into these it disappears; even among these it shows itself again. The body is made of the five tatwas; the five tatwas exist therein in the subtle form. They are known by the learned who devote themselves to the tatwas".

"On this account I shall speak of the rise of breath in the body; by knowing the nature of inspiration and expiration comes into being the knowledge of the three times (past, present and future) ; omniscience is caused by it if well understood. Whoever knows the analysis of the Nadis and the Prana, the analysis of the tatwas and the analysis of the conjunctive sushumna gets salvation " (release from re-births).

The other fruits of such knowledge are: the power to kill enemies; to form friendships; to acquire wealth, comfort and reputation; to control the sex of offspring; to get access to a king; to get a king into one's power; to propititiate gods; the power of locomotion and of the exercise of bodily functions; exemption from being controlled by the heavenly bodies; ability to lengthen and shorten the limbs at will; fulfillment of desires; victory; cheating time; great bliss and godlike power; the statement closing with: "He who has the knowledge of breath in his head has fortune at his feet. " The method of using the knowledge to obtain the fruits consists largely in commencing undertakings at such times as are known to be propitious by the movement of the tatwas in the body. Here the breath of the lungs plays its part, but, for all that is told, only as an indicator of the tatwic movements, as conduits of which the Ida, Pingala and Sushumna have their importance. Divination is accomplished by means of a like knowledge of tatwic movement, and rules for practicing it fill a large part of the book.

Each of the tatwas is known to the yogi by its color, form, taste and mode of vibration, the power to discern which is in each case to be acquired by an appropriate practice. Except that concentration of the mind is never forgotten and that in the end one of the Kumbhakas is recommended, the yoga methods of the little book are unlike any that have heretofore been cited. The most important of them is given in the following, under the heading of " Meditation of the Tatwas and mastery over them " : " But now we are going to explain the most important and final mode of practicing. This is the secret which the sages of India only were acquainted with, and up to this time was only a legacy to the most promising and perfect adept of yoga. The beginner at first will think it a mere joke and perhaps madness. But a short practice will fully assure him of the important results to be gained by the practice. He will by degrees become powerful enough to have at his will all the visible worlds before his inward eyes and command the secrets of nature".

" During the day, when the sky is clear, let him once or twice for about an hour or two draw his mind from all external things, and sitting on an easy chair let him fix his eyes on any particular part of the blue sky and go on looking at it without allowing them to twinkle".

"At first he will see the waves of the water which surrounds the whole world".

"Some days after, as the eye becomes practiced, he will see different sorts of buildings, etc., in the air, and many other wonderful things, too. When the neophyte reaches this stage of practice he should be sure of gaining success".

"After this he will see different sorts of mixed colors of the Tatwas in the sky which will, after a constant and resolute practice, show themselves in their respective colors. To test the truth of which, the neophyte, during the practice, should occasionally close his eyes and compare the color floating in the sky with that he sees inwardly. When both are the same the operation is right. Other wonders resulting from this will present themselves to the yogi. This practice is to be done in the day time, "

" For the night he must sit with his shin bones to the ground, letting his feet touch his calves; put his hands upon his knees, having the fingers pointed towards his body; then fix his eyes on the tip of his nose, and meditate upon his breath going in and coming out". At this stage of perfection the yogi should commence as follows:

" Getting up at two or three a.m., let him now fix his mind on the Tatwa then in course (in his body). If the Tatwa in course is then Prithivi (the earth), let him think of it as something having four corners (the earth in scriptural times was always square), having a good yellow color, sweet smelling, small in body, and taking away all diseases. Let him at the same time repeat the word Lam. It is very easy to imagine such a thing".

After giving a like sort of formula for each of the other four Tatwas, each closing with a magic word of one syllable, the book goes on to say: "By diligent practice these syllables, uttered by the tongue of a yogi, become inseparable from the Tatwa. Whenever he repeats any of these the special Tatwa appears with as much force as he may will ; and thus it is that a yogi can cause, whenever he likes, lightning, rain, hurricanes, etc". By the mastery over the Tatwas thus obtained, he can also compel the right one to move in the right time and place, so as to become auspicious to any proposed undertaking (as one would regulate the wind by means of the weathercock).

The work of Swatmaram is no doubt very old, but this little book must be much older, if we may judge by its secular, non-devotional character, the absence of metaphysics, its primitive rules for divination and the large space they occupy, its having been of late laid away and nearly lost, as the preface to the translation indicates, and, finally, by the marks it bears of having been expurgated in the interest of modesty.

Karma Yoga., or the Yoga of Work

Although seclusion and leisure are so important in the practice of yoga as almost to be conditions essential to it, yet men have lived who, in spite of the distractions of active life in the world, have attained to some degree of it at least, as, for example, Plotinus; and both Hindu and Chinese writers tell of others, legendary or supposititious, to whom the very occupations which would ordinarily disturb mental concentration have served as objects on which to exercise it. The Swami Vivekananda, who in one of his eight lectures on Karma Yoga goes so far as to say : " Just by work men can get where Buddha got by meditation and Christ by prayer", in another tells of a poor, hard-working woman who, having read the thoughts of a young Sanyasi, or monk, in a way that so astonished him that he fell at her feet and exclaimed: "Mother, how did you know that?" answered him: " Boy, I do not know your yoga or your practices, but all my life I have struggled to do my duty; that is all the yoga I practice, and by doing my duty I have become illumined". She then referred him to a butcher as one whose gifts, acquired in the midst of his heavy labors, were much above her own, and who afterwards, in an interval of those labors, sat down and gave the same monk a lecture, which is now a celebrated book in India. When it was finished the hearer could not but ask : ' ' Why are you in a butcher's body and doing such filthy, ugly work ?" to which the reply was: "I neither know your yoga, nor have I become a Sanyasi; never went out of the world nor into the forest, but all this has come to me through doing my duty in my position". Notwithstanding the prominence given to duty in this narration, it would be wrong to thence infer that the fruits of yoga are bestowed as rewards for the performance of duty; to assume that they are given as prizes to encourage the doing of good acts to others would be to go counter to the whole tenor of yoga teaching, which relates only to one's dealings with one's self as a means of arriving at his very self. What brought illumination to the woman and man just referred to must be presumed to have been doing the work which duty required of them with concentrated minds. Concentration itself being the operative means and the object concentrated on being of small moment, it might be possible for a strong mind to direct itself so intently on even manual labor as to obtain the Siddhis as immediate, and deliverance as ultimate results.

The Chinese sage, Chuang-Tzu, tells a story of which another cutter-up of meat is the hero, thus: "Prince Hui's cook was cutting up a bullock. Every blow of his hand, every heave of his shoulders, every tread of his foot, every thrust of his knee, every whshh of rent flesh, every chhk of the chopper, was in perfect harmony — rythmical like the dance of the mulberry grove, simultaneous like the chords of Ching Shou. " " Well done", cried the Prince; "yours is skill indeed". "Sire", replied the cook, "I have always devoted myself to Tao (which here means the same as yoga). It is better than skill. When I first began to cut up bullocks I saw before me simply whole bullocks. After three years' practice I saw no more whole animals. And now I work with my mind and not with my eye. When my senses bid me stop, but my mind urges me on, I fall back upon eternal principles. I follow such openings or cavities as there may be, according to the natural constitution of the animal. A good cook changes his chopper once a year, because he cuts. An ordinary cook once a month — because he hacks. But I have had this chopper nineteen years, and although I have cut up many thousand bullocks, its edge is as if fresh from the whetstone". Another narration of the same sage not only illustrates the point that common labor may serve the purpose of mental concentration, and thereby as above develop something "better than skill", but also explains, so far as it is explicable, the difference between knowledge such as can be taught in words, and one branch at least of such as comes by yoga practice, the one being communicable by a few hours of instruction and the other obtainable only by years of practice, in which hand and head cooperate to give a mastery which is beyond knowledge. An old wheelwright, who undertakes to explain to his prince the difference in question, is made to say :

"Let me take an illustration from my own trade. In making a wheel, if you work too slowly, you can't make it firm; if you work too fast the spokes won't fit in. You must neither go too slowly nor too fast. There must be co-ordination of mind and hand. Words cannot explain what it is, but there is some mysterious art therein. I cannot teach it to my son ; nor can he learn it from me. Consequently, though seventy years old, I am still making wheels in my old age". May not that something slowly acquired by co-ordination of mind and hand, in which the ability of the artisan and artist lies, be indeed a kind of yoga ? May not artistic inspiration be as much the product of artistic labor as the yogis' enlightenment is of the yoga practice ?

It was to be expected that the practical Chinese would put yoga to mundane uses, and accordingly the writings of Chuang-Tzu are illustrated with many more instances of like bearing with the above; of these one more will be quoted: "The man who forged swords for the Minister of War was eighty years of age, yet he never made the slightest slip in his work".

The Minister of War said to him, "Is it your skill, Sir, or have you any method?"

" It is concentration, " replied the man. "When twenty years old I took to forging swords. If a thing was not a sword, I did not notice it. I availed myself of whatever energy I did not use in other directions in order to secure greater efficiency in the direction required. Still more of that which is never without use — Tao (yoga). So that there was nothing which did not lend its aid".

The Japanese armorers, too, it is said, when they undertake to forge a blade of superior quality, call in the aid of yoga concentration, but in a more ceremonious manner, hammering away in a state of true spiritual exaltation. And the methods of these craftsmen are none the less true yoga practice for the object concentrated on being the work presently in hand and the fruit of it merely earthly profit and advantage. Of course it is not here intended to include in the same category with this handicraft inspiration the higher kinds of knowledge that come in Samadhi.

We have seen in what has been thus far disclosed of Hindu yoga practice that the concentration of the mind required by it may be upon any one thing or thought, point, place, word, act, or nothing at all — absolute void, the last the best of all. Also that yoga may be efficiently practiced in the household or the forest, in solitude, or crowds, though, doubtless, seclusion and solitude, and exemption from physical labor, furnish by far the better conditions. But the range of concentration may be still further extended; it may include bodily sensations and mental emotions. Intense pain or intense pleasure of mind or body have power to command the attention. One office of pain in the scheme of Nature may be to concentrate the mental powers on the injury or disorder, of which it is the effect and the outcry, with curative force, and the common fainting fit may be but a form of trance, Samadhi, brought on by intensity of the agony, alarm or grief. The " witches' sleep", which so often came to the sufferers on the rack or at the stake, and which is said by some to have saved Servetus at the last from feeling the full measure of Calvin's hate, may have been brought on by concentration on this or that subject or thing, but more likely was induced by a powerful focussing of the mental faculties on the bodily agony then and there being undergone or impending, for if the witches were really witches they were "sensitive" and easily put into a trance, just as Boehme was, who went into one at the sight of a point of light on a newly scoured pewter platter, or John of the Cross, in whose presence, in his latter days, it would not do to sing a verse lest he should immediately lose consciousness and rise and float in the air. Faintings connected with joyful sensations of any kind can hardly be attributed to concentration on anything else than the joy presently felt. There is a yoga practice in India based on sexual love, and it has two branches, termed of the right and left hand.

Some Concluding Remarks on Hindu Yoga

Of the 275 sections composing that part of Swatmaram's manual that treats of Hatha Yoga, there are only three that mention release or deliverance, and these being out of joint with all the 272 others must be considered as having got into the compilation — which is all the book claims to be — without right. The little work on "The Science of Breath " is entirely bare of any promise of, or allusion to, any other than worldly benefits to be enjoyed in this life as the reward of the neophyte's practice, while that reward is distinctly stated to be the qualifying him as a magician with the powers usually accorded to such, besides others usually attributed only to gods, together with the enjoyment of "immeasurable bliss". Both works relate evidently to the primitive, unsophisticated yoga of the times when the Rig Vedas, quite as exclusively mundane in the benefits they promise, were composed by the earliest yogis, and when the Brahmans were not as yet a caste, but merely a body of household priests and practical magicians working for hire. But when the great and wonderful secret doctrine, born of the brains of the Kshatrya class, of other and superior blood to these, and elaborated to perfection while years by centuries rolled on, was at length made known and a new philosophy given to the world, the old magic was put to a new use, and as indicating its new end and aim, which was that of escaping from re-birth through junction with the first principle of all things, took the name of Yoga; and because it was the gift of the warrior class, from which the rulers of the people were chosen, became distinctively known as Rajah, or Royal Yoga, while the other kept that which expresses its method and not its object, namely, Ha Tha, or Breath Yoga. Yet there are some who think Rajah Yoga means only royal road, i.e. easy road.

The way in which the long-kept secret got out is narrated in the Upanishads, thus: A priest said to his son, " Shvetaketu, go dwell as a Brahman student, for none of our family was ever unlearned, a mere hanger-on of Brahmanhood". Then Shvetaketu, going when he was twelve years old, returned when he was twenty-four, after studying all the Vedas, conceited, vain of his learning, and proud.

His father then sent him to the Court of King Pravahanna, who, addressing him, said:

"Youth, has thy father instructed thee? "

"Yes, sire", replied the young Brahman. Then the King asked him: " Knowest thou whither go those who die out of this world? "

" No", he replied.

" Knowest thou how they return again? "

" No", he replied.

" Knowest thou the turning apart of the two ways?" (the way of the gods and the way of the fathers).

" No", he replied.

" Knowest thou why that world is not overfilled? "

" No", he replied.

"Knowest thou how, at the fifth offering, the waters take human voice?"

" No", he replied.

" Then how saidst thou that thou hast received the teaching? For how is he taught who knows not these things? "

The youth thereupon goes and reports his discomfiture to his father, but refuses to go again to the King to be taught, so the old man goes alone and begs for instruction. The King, after telling him: " Never before thee did this teaching reach the Brahmans, but among all peoples it was the hereditary instruction of the Kshatryas alone", granted his request.

Be this story itself true or not, it well enough conveys the truth that subsequently to the giving out of the Vedic Revelations there had grown up in secret quite another doctrine of life, death and immortality from what they convey, that was, after a very long period, in some way given to the world, or to the priesthood rather, who had lent no hand in its making up, and who, though ostensibly accepting, paid little regard to it. The unanswered questions of the King imply that it contained : (1), A modified world of spirits, consisting of a land of the fathers and a land of the gods, with a special way to each, but only a temporary sojourn in either; (2), Rebirth; (3), Release from it, and final absorption in Brahman.

As to the peculiar Hindu belief in absorption, it may be conceived of as arising from the acquisition of magical powers, always esteemed to be god-like, in connection with the subjective experiences that come with them, among which are certain blissful sensations, that might well suggest to the practicer's mind that he was losing his every-day self in something. We have seen that yoga literature claims for practicers who attain to yoga power to work as good miracles as any god. This being so, it would be natural for the attainer, as one by one miraculous powers came to him, to think himself on the way to become God, and when Samadhi, with its bliss, illumination and sinking of the outer conscious in the inner one was finally reached, that he should exclaim, " I am Brahman !" Thus the idea of absorption may very well have arisen from the wonderful experiences of yoga practice. But it is more than probable that before this idea was reached that of absorption in inferior deities had its place, for those came first in order of time, but naturally, also, this lower conception would give place to the higher one now become the core of the Vedanta philosophy and leave no trace in Hindu literature. So much for the belief in absorption. But how came we by the doctrine of re-births ? Mr, Charles Johnston, in the "Metaphysical Magazine" for May, 1896, refers it to an intuition. He says: " The early Kshatrya teaching was an intuition of the potency of the moral and spiritual forces as the determining powers in life and a belief in re-birth as the natural outcome of the reality and continuance of those energies". Thus a scholar, apparently well read in Hindu learning, has found there no more solid reason for this very solidly fixed belief than an inference drawn from an intuition.

When King Pravahanna gave out the long-hidden Rajah Philosophy, there came with it no special Rajah Yoga, but in the course of time difference in purpose brought difference in method, and the old system of training for the development of magicians through intent, persistent, not thinking, aided by certain bodily acts efficient to arrest thought, gradually grew into the seemingly more intellectual and spiritual one now most in vogue, of scorning physical means and magical ends and agonizing in the hardest kind of metaphysical thinking for the purpose of getting to God.

Sankaracharya says : "One who desires knowledge for final absolution must set himself seriously to think".

"Knowledge is not produced by any means other than right thinking; just as the objects in the universe are never perceived but by the help of light".

"Who am I ? How is this evolved? Who is its creator ? What is the material of which it is made ? This is the form of rational thought".

And then the young philosopher goes on rather dogmatically to tell the disciple what to think.

If more were known of the yogas other than Hindu more resemblance might be found between them and it than appears when the above condensation which the richness of the literature relating to it has rendered possible is compared with the more meagre accounts concerning the others with which we shall have to be content. But as it is certain important features of the one will be found to be wanting in all others. The positions, breathings, movements and listenings, in short, all of importance in Swatmaram's book, save simple mental concentration, is peculiar to the Hindu practice. In other words, all that distinguishes Hatha from other Hindu yogas also distinguishes Hindu Yoga as a whole from all others. Again, though in some of those others union with God in some mode is held up as the object to be attained by the practice, such union never amounts to absorption, nor effects release from re-births. Whatever other reward may attend any other than the Hindu practicer's labors, it is not the getting out of life — the shaking off of this troublesome universe.

It is true that Hindu Yoga calls itself a religion, and that it utilizes religious belief and emotion as means of concentration, but otherwise it is peculiar among religions in denying that either of them is essential to yoga practice, or even an aid to it, save for people whose minds are able to hold such beliefs and are of temperaments too emotional to do without them. The Christian yogi must remain a devotee till he dies; the Hindu, if he ever were one, is rid of all the burthens of religion as soon as he has "attained " ; an atheist will do just as well as any other to make a yogi of. If of philosophical tastes he may concentrate on logical propositions, and this is Gnana Yoga. If of mystical tendencies he may study the stirring within him of the faculties of his own soul aroused to movement by the stilling of his mind, and this is Rajah Yoga. Or if he be a man of work, he may put his attention fixedly on what he has to do, and this is Karma Yoga, But whatever the method be called, it is well worth notice that the expositors of it are careful to stir in with the concentration more or less of Pranyama, breathing. Thus mental concentration and physical breathing are inseparable companions in every form of Hindu Yoga. Concentration is in all others, but breathing is absent. Now, there are facts which seem to show that this difference is of the greatest importance; among which are these: that the breathing is proved to have power to still the mind, as, indeed, every one may test for himself, and that the late American experiments prove that concentration undertaken solely for the purpose of so stilling the mind can also set up the breathings in an involuntary manner, as well as the Mudras and other bodily movements, internal and external, which the manuals of Hatha Yoga direct to be voluntarily done.

CHAPTER XVIII - CHINESE YOGA

When, three centuries before Christ, Buddhism carried with it into China Hindu Yoga, it found there something much older than itself called Tao whose scriptures, embodied in the "Tao-Te-King", or" The Book of the Way and of Virtue", attributed to the sage Lao-Tsee, who lived three centuries earlier still, though supposed by scholars to be spurious in part and in large part incomplete, is nevertheless the authoritative exposition of the old Taoism which Confucius came to disturb and the recognized authority of the new and corrupted cult of that name.

Old Taoism never had a personal god; the persons of its mythology were not gods, and the gods of its philosophy were not persons. The "supreme magistrate" whom the book in question in one place mentions, was merely a spirit who, acting upon information brought to him by other spirits who went up and down in the earth doing duty as detectives, rewarded and punished according to desert both the living and the dead. In another place a "supreme master of heaven" is alluded to as "coming subsequent to Tao", and in other literature an "emperor of heaven" and again a "king of heaven" are named; but these bore rule in heaven only and their jurisdiction did not interfere with that of the one heaven-ordained ruler of all the earth, namely, the Emperor of China. Of philosophical gods, there were three, but they were like the Brahman of the Hindu philosophy, primordial principles only, high above worship, obedience and love, and nothing like the trinity, made up of Brahman endowed with personality and sex and his associates personal Vichnu and Siva, nor that of the Egyptians, which was simply a holy family made up of Osiris, the father, Isis, the mother, and Horus, their son; nor yet that of the Christians, which was modeled on this last, except that in deference to the contempt felt generally throughout early Christendom for her sex, the Virgin Mary was left out, and the Holy Spirit, till then unknown as a god, put in her place. Which was a sad mistake, for the amended god-head was so inartificially put together that long and horrible wars resulting from efforts to understand it have left it still incomprehensible to the mortal mind, while, so far as history relates, no bloodshed at all had to be invoked in explanation of its prototype, the simple family circle of Egypt.

The construction of the Christian trinity, according to Saint Augustine, is as follows: "We say, we do, that the father is the father of the son, and that the son is the son of the father, and that the holy spirit is the spirit of the father and the son, without being either the father or the son". Thus the Holy Ghost, who as everybody knows begat the son, is declared to have done so before he himself had existence, since as the spirit of his child he could not have had being in advance of that child.

Much prettier word-work are the expositions of the only two impersonal trinities of which there is record, namely that of Old Taoism, made by Lao-Tsee and that of the Neoplatonists, made by Plotinus, the parallelism of which is the more remarkable when it is considered that however much the Greeks may have learned from India, the literature of China must have been quite beyond their reach. Here is a statement of each, member by member, that of Plotinus being from the hand of M. Bouillet, his translator and editor:

" The foundation of the whole system of Plotinus is the theory of the three hypostatic principles, that is to say, of the three Divine principles which from all eternity have emanated the one from the other". The first is called " the First", " the Good'" because all depends on it, all aspires to it, all hold of it existence, life and thought. It is also called " the One", " the Simple", "the Absolute", which has manifested its power in producing all intelligible beings. (But what he thus indicates Plotinus expressly says cannot be named.)

Now turning to the Tao-Te-King we read: "Tao produced One", "One produced Two", "Two produced Three", " Three have produced all beings". Also: "The being without a name is the origin of heaven and earth; with a name it is the mother of all things". " Tao is vague, confused". " Tao is void but exhaustless, profound, the patriarch of all beings; pure, subsisting eternally". " Tao is beyond sense, eternal, nameless, formless, rooted in non-being, obscure, without color or sound, cannot be touched, is incorporeal, form without form, image without image".

The second member of the Neoplatonic trinity is thus described: "The second principle is Intelligence, which embraces in its universality all the individual intelligences. In thinking itself, Intelligence possesses all things; it is all things, because in it the thinking subject, the object thought of and the thought itself are identical". "Its ideas are the pure forms, types of all that exists here below in the world of sense, the essences, the real beings, the intelligibles ; they compose the intelligible world".

In the Tao-Te-King we read: "The visible forms of the great Virtue (Te) emanate from Tao solely". "Within it are images". "Within it are beings". "Within it is a spiritual essence, and that essence is profoundly true".

The third member of the Neoplatonic trinity is thus described: "The third principle is the universal soul, or the soul of the world, from which proceed all the individual souls". " There are two parts to it, the principal power of the soul, or the celestial soul, which contemplates ntelligence and thence receives its forms, and the inferior power of the soul, called natural and generative power, total Reason of the Universe, because it transmits to matter the seminal reasons which fashion and form the animals".

145

The Tao-Te-King says: " It, Tao, can be regarded as the mother of the Universe". " It is spread throughout the Universe " (note 8). "There is not a creature that does not possess it". " Tao flows everywhere". "All beings rely on it to give them birth, and it repels none". "It loves and sustains all beings". "It is able to give aid to them and conduct them to perfection". "Tao produces beings, Virtue (Te) sustains them. They manifest them under a material form, and perfect them by a forcible secret impulsion". " Tao produces beings, sustains and causes them to grow, perfects them, feeds them, protects them". " That which is void, non-being, immaterial, is called Tao, or the way; that which transforms and sustains all creatures is Te, or Virtue". " An immaterial breath forms Harmony". Readers who will carefully compare these Chinese and Greek triads will find their parallelism so close that they must wonder that lines so far apart in time and space, the one projected from the Chinese and the other from the Greek intellect, could run so nearly, if not exactly, equi-distant at every point as these do.

Like Plotinus, who declares the first principle of his trinity to be too great for a name, and uses the terms "the One", "the First", "the Good", "the Simple", " the Absolute", to point at what he may not name. Lao-Tse uses the vague word Tao to indicate his first and ineffable principle, "the being without a name". To his life-giving, life-sustaining principle, corresponding to the universal soul of Plotinus, and which must be ranked as third in order, he applies the name Virtue (Te), but has none for that intermediate one corresponding to the Neoplatonist's " Intelligence "; for it " Tao " has again to serve, as it does for numberless other things and nothings — in short, for whatever is beyond reach of normal consciousness, and all within its reach that relates to what is so beyond it.

Not only has this old Taoism a superior godhead, if so it may be called, but it has a moral ideal that transcends all others, and which even Neoplatonism cannot match, an ideal that is above justice, above humanity, above virtue. The eighteenth chapter of the Tao-Te-King reads:

"When the Great Way had decayed, humanity and justice made their appearance".

"When the family ceased to line in good harmony, acts of filial piety and paternal affection became known".

"When states fell into disorder, faithful and devoted subjects came into notice".

The thirty-eighth chapter reads:

" Men of superior virtue ignore their virtue; and that is why they have virtue".

" Men of inferior virtue never forget their virtue ; that is why they have no virtue".

" Men of superior virtue practice it without dreaming of it".

" Men of inferior virtue practice it with intention".

" Men of superior humanity practice it without dreaming of it".

" Men of superior equity practice it with intention".

" Men of superior urbanity practice it and nobody responds to it; then they use violence to obtain return payment of it".

"This is why one can have virtue after having lost Tao; humanity after having lost virtue; equity after having lost humanity ; urbanity after having lost equity".

" Urbanity is but the husk of rectitude and of sincerity; it is the source of disorder".

Jesus of Nazareth when he taught that men should return good for evil went no further in his altruism than Lao-Tsee had already gone when he declared that they should "avenge injuries with benefits"; which latter saying when reported to Confucius he criticised by the question: "With what then would you return good ? " We of these days so remote from the supposed Golden Age to which the old Taoists looked back as to a paradise lost but yet possible to be regained, will be disposed to accept the criticism, but in the times when it was uttered it may have seemed harsh and unwise to many. The Tao-Te-King anticipates Plato in asserting the metaphysical principle that contraries mutually produce each other. It contains many prudential maxims for ruling every-day life and political maxims for ruling the state, the latter conveying doctrine sadly needed in these our days of over-governing, and which are intensified in these two sententious aphorisms: "Who rules ruins", "To rule men and serve heaven nothing is comparable to moderation". Capital punishment is declared to be not only wrong, but ineffectual. No personal God is mentioned, no devotional observance enjoined save that ancestor worship is alluded to as any other existing custom might be. In like way spiritual beings are mentioned, but they are mostly terrestrial demons. Further than this there is nothing said of creed or rite, temple, shrine or priest, future rewards or punishments, or in fact of any "future state" at all.

Old Taoism was not pessimistic any more than old Hinduism was in the times when length of life and not release from it was the thing most desired, and good crops, full udders and fat calves were prayed for rather than spiritual gifts. Tao was practiced for what Hindu yogis scorn and spurn as obstructions in their path, namely, the siddhis, or miraculous powers, the siddhi chiefly prized, so far as the Tao-Te-King reveals, being the ability to rule a state, which ability seems to have lain as much in a certain magic power to influence the conduct of men as in the political wisdom that was supposed to be also a gift of Tao. Rulers of Ancient China have carried their belief in these gifts so far that it was as common for them to call to their aid to serve as ministers of state, governors of provinces and officials of other kinds, hermits from the woods and caves, as it has been for British sovereigns to call to their aid members of the landed aristocracy. And, more than that, in comparatively recent times two of the Chinese emperors have actually made experiments in governing their subjects without any resort to force. An experiment of the opposite sort was that of state communism tried during some twenty years, but with such poor success that no repetition of it has been attempted. The following is a synopsis of what the Tao-Te-King affirms Tao to be, to make which complete there has had to be a few repetitions of what went before:

" Tao is a being; the first principle; being that is between heaven and earth; void, but exhaustless; the patriarch of all beings, veils its subtlety and tempers its splendor and assimilates itself to dust; seems to subsist eternally; its parentage unknown; seems to have preceded the ' master of heaven ' ; is beyond sense ; eternal ; nameless; formless; re-entering into non-being; vague; indetermined; confused; contains images; contains beings; is profound; is obscure; has a spiritual essence which is profoundly true; contains an infallible witness (of itself) ; has a name that never fails; gives birth to all beings ; existed before the heavens and the earth ; is calm, is immaterial; circulates everywhere without danger; can be regarded as the mother of the universe; has no name, but may be called Tao (Way) ; is grand, fugacious, remote; returning; is little, but the whole world cannot conquer it; gives power over all things to those who have it; as soon as it was divided it took a name; it is spread throughout the universe; all beings return to it as rivers to seas ; it extends in all directions ; there is not a creature, animal or plant that does not possess it; all beings rely on it to give them birth, and it repels none; it loves and nourishes all beings, and regards not itself as their master ; is without desires ; all beings submit themselves to it ; its movement is produced by return to non-being ; to be weak is the function of Tao; it conducts beings to perfection; is a great square of which the angles are not seen ; a great vase which seems far from being finished; a great voice of which the sound is imperceptible; a great image of whom the form is not seen; produces beings which Te (virtue) nourishes; and to which the two give bodies, which they perfect by a secret forcible impulsion; Tao nourishes beings; makes them to grow; feeds them, protects them; produces without appropriating them, nor takes glory to itself; reigns over but leaves them free; behold a profound goodness ! Tao was the principle of the world and has become its mother; it should be cultivated by all; evil spirits, however powerful, do no harm in a kingdom governed by Tao ; it is the asylum of all beings ; the treasure of the virtuous man and the support of the wicked one ; is found naturally, without searching all day for it; by it the guilty obtain liberty and life".

Let the reader now, bearing in mind what has been before particularized concerning the Hindu yogis, compare it with the following detailsquoted from the Tao-Te-King :

"The saint makes it his business to do nothing, and his instructions to consist in silence ; the saint withdraws himself from his body, and his body preserves itself; has no private interests; keeps down his desires; casts off all desires; practices non-action ; occupies himself with nonoccupation ; does not fail, because he does not act ; makes his desires consist in the absence of all desire, and his studies to consist in the absence of all study; fears glory as he would shame; his body weighs on him as a great calamity; without leaving his house he knows the Universe; gets where he wants to be without taking a step; can name objects without seeing them; without acting accomplishes great things; he is careful of his body, and economizes his vital forces; he who knows Tao is not learned; he who is learned knows not Tao; the sage is best pleased in a lowly dwelling, remote from the crowd; in ancient times those who excelled in practicing Tao were shrewd, subtle, abstracted, penetrating, profound beyond fathoming; were timid, irresolute, shunning observation, grave, of rude exterior, empty as a valley, stupid in appearance; the sage by a profound calm gradually grows in spirituality; is in no danger from man or beast; is exempt from death; he shuts his mouth, closes his ears and eyes, represses his activity, releases himself of all ties, tempers his interior light, assimilates himself to the vulgar; he attaches himself to nothing, and therefore loses nothing; goes poorly clad; only he who is constantly exempt from passions can see his own spiritual essence; there is no greater crime than to deliver yourself over to your desires, no greater misfortune than not to know how to be sufficient unto yourself, no greater calamity than the desire of gain; if the man preserves unity his soul and body may remain indissoluble".

Chuang-Tzu

An examination into old Taoism that should neglect the writings of Chuang-Tzü, the great disciple of Lao-Tsee, who lived three hundred years later than his master, would be incomplete. He was more than a disciple, for besides amplifying his teacher's work, he covered much new ground, being as bold an originator as he was a clear expositor. He made an impression on the minds of his countrymen that has endured till this day, although one of his commentators says that none exists capable of understanding him, and he himself said he would never be understood.

Here are a few passages from writings attributed to him, Giles' translation:

"At the beginning of the beginning even nothing did not exist. Then came the period of the nameless". "Let knowledge stop at the unknowable". " There is nothing on earth that does not rise and fall, but nothing ever perishes altogether».

"To put yourself in subjective relations with externals, without consciousness of their objectivity, recognizing that all things are One — that is Tao".

Subjective Results of Tao Attainment

"But man can attain to formlessness and vanquish death. Man may abide in the everlasting. He may bring nature to a condition of One".

"One who extends his sway over heaven and earth and influences all things, and who, lodging within the confines of a body with its channels of sight and sound, brings his knowledge to know that all things are One, and that his soul endures forever".

" He who knows what God is and knows what man is has attained. Knowing what God is, he knows that he himself proceeded from thence".

"Cherish that which is within you, and shut off that which is without, for much learning is a curse. Then I will place you upon that abode of great light which is the source of the positive power, and escort you through the gate of profound mystery, which is the source of the negative power. These powers are the controllers of heaven and earth, and each contains the other".

The Lesser Siddhis .

The Taoist sages had power to transform themselves to the eyes of others. Thus Hu Tzü, when a famous magician came to see him, showed himself first as decrepit and near to death, next as having still some recuperative power left, next as in full health, and lastly "as Tao appeared before time was", whereupon the visitor ran away in terror. Of this magician it is said that "He knew all about birth and death, loss and gain, misfortune and happiness, long life and short life — predicting events to a day with supernatural accuracy".

Now, gifts like these last were also possessed by the sages, but were for some reason contemned by Lao-Tsee, who calls them "false knowledge, which is but the flower of Tao and the principle of ignorance", reminding us of the yogis contempt for all the siddhis, including what the Taoist saints accepted as well as what they rejected. And yet the very book in which he wrote this was saved from the general burning (ordered by a certain emperor, in order to start history afresh with his reign) only because it was a book of divination.

Tao Practice

Though ancient Taoism has left no manual of practice such as ancient Yoga has, the following from Chuang-Tzü seem to recognize that a system of practice existed and that time was an important element of it. He says:

" Preserve your form complete and your vitality secure. Let no anxious thoughts intrude. And then in three years you may attain to this".

" One year after receiving your instructions I became naturally simple. After two years I could adapt myself as required. After three years I understood. After four years my intelligence developed. After five years it was complete. After six years the spirit entered into me. After seven I knew God. After eight life and death existed for me no more. After nine, perfection".

The following, however, seems to imply that for " the right sort of man " there is a short cut to attainment, and by methods which, if disclosed, would suggest the most mysterious of the Yoga madras, the Vajroli.

Nan Po Tzu Kuei said to Nii Yii, by one authority said to be a woman ; " You are old, but your countenance is like that of a child. How is this ? "

Nii Yii replied: "I have learned Tao".

" Could I get it by studying ? " asked the other.

" I fear not", said Nii Yii. " You are not the sort of a man. There was Pu Laing I. He had all the qualifications of a sage, but not Tao. Now I had Tao, though none of the qualifications. But do you imagine that much as I wished it I was able to teach Tao to him so that he could be a perfect sage ? Had it been so, then to teach Tao to one who has the qualifications of a sage would be an easy matter. No, sir. I imparted it to him as though withholding; and in three days for him this sublunary state had ceased to exist. When he had attained to this, I withheld again; and in seven days more the external world had ceased to be. And so again for another nine days, when he became unconscious of his own existence. He became etherealized, next possessed of perfect wisdom, then without past or present, and finally able to enter there where life and death are no more — where killing does not take away life, nor does prolongation of life add to the duration of existence. In that state he is ever in accord with the exigencies of his environment; and this is to be battered but not bruised. And he who can be thus battered but not bruised is on his way to perfection". " And how did you manage to get hold of all this ? " asked the other.

"I got it from books", replied Nii Yii; "and the books got it from learning, and learning from investigation, and investigation from co-ordination, and co-ordination from application, and application from desire to know, and desire to know from the unknown, and the unknown from the great void, and the great void from infinity! "

CHAPTER XIX - EGYPTIAN YOGA

The earliest records of the religion of Egypt tell of a very philosophically conceived god, without beginning or end. The sole progenitor in heaven and earth, uncreated and self-begotten. "But", says Mr. Lenorment, "this sublime notion, if it was retained in the esoteric doctrine, soon became obscured and disfigured by the conceptions of the priests and the ignorance of the people". The exoteric notions, which prevailed over it, had to do with secondary and personal deities only, and Egyptian magic occupied itself merely with the hosts of these. They were ruled over by a god in chief, it is true, but he was one of their own sort, being like Jehovah, a promoted tutelary divinity. At each of the many removals of the capital city from the lower valley of the Nile in the direction of its source, from time to time made necessary by the shifting that way of the centre of population, a new god in chief had to be installed, since the custom of the country made the local deity of the district ex-officio Lord of the Universe. Here there was no Brahman into which souls could be absorbed. Nor did the Egyptian religion, though including belief in rebirths, allow any means of escape from them by absorption in any god, high or low, or in fact in any mode whatever.

Yet Egypt had a yoga, and one which, like all others, was only attainable through rigorous self-discipline, which, acting on the very nature of the practicer, transformed him into a magician. It amounted to a junction, and a junction with a god. All magical work was esteemed to be no more nor no less than god-work. What a god could do a magician could, and what a magician could do a god could. Thus, just as in the case of the Hindu idea of absorption in Brahman, that of assimilation with a secondary divinity would naturally arise in the Egyptian magician's conceit, as one by one he acquired, by his efforts and patience, god-like powers, while the blissful experiences underwent, together with the bewildering sensations of the trance, always incident to yoga practice, would aid the illusion.

Mr. Lenorment says: "There was, indeed, a formal belief in ancient Egypt, which was attested by numerous passages from the religious texts, that the knowledge of divine things elevated a man to the heights of the gods, identified him with them, and ended by blending his substance with that of the divine. The primary idea of all the magic formula which were designed to repel the torments of life and the attacks of venomous animals was always assimilation to the gods. The virtue of the formula lay not in an invocation of the divine power, but in the fact of a man's proclaiming himself such or such a god, and when he, in pronouncing the incantation, called to his aid any one of the various members of the Egyptian Pantheon, it was as one of themselves that he had a right to the assistance of his companions". And he quotes an incantation in which the magician is made to say:

" Do not be against me ! I am Amen.

" I am Anhur, the good guardian.

'* I am the great master of the sword.

"Do not erect thyself ! I am Mouth.

" Do not try to surprise me ! I am Set.

" Do not raise thy two arms against me ! I am Sothis.

"Do not seize me ! I am Sethu".

Such was Egyptian yoga, or theurgry, as the Neoplatonists named it.

Concerning the methods of practice, Mr, Lenorment, as just seen, leaves it to be inferred that it consisted in "the knowledge of divine things", but in a quotation he gives from the ritual of the dead there is more than a hint that in Egypt, as elsewhere, steadfast concentration was the key to that knowledge, with austerities for aids and trance for incident. It is this: " This chapter was found at Seaenou, written in blue, upon a cube of bloodstone under the feet of a great god; it was found in the days of King Mycerinus, the veracious, by the royal son Hartatef, when he was travelling to inspect the accounts of the temples. He repeated a hymn to himself, after which he went into ecstasies. He took it away in the King's chariots as soon as he saw what was written upon it. It is a great mystery. One sees and hears nothing else while reciting this pure and holy chapter. Never again approach a woman; eat neither meat or fish".

A very full exposition of Egyptian magic is found in the celebrated reply of Jamblichus, the neoplatonist, to a letter written by Porphery as if to a priest of Egypt, making enquiries about the religion of that country, in which reply it is strenuously argued that magical works are performed by divine and not by human power, and that to attain to that state of union with the gods by means of which their abilities may be appropriated for the benefit of men, philosophical thought is of no value, but only theurgic work. He says, concerning this last: "For a conception of the mind does not conjoin theurgists with the gods; since if this were the case what would hinder those who philosophize theoretically from having a theurgic union with the gods ? Now, however, in reality this is not the case. For the perfect efficacy of ineffable works, which are divinely performed in a way surpassing all intelligence, and the power of inexplicable symbols, which are known only to the gods, impart theurgic union. Hence we do not perform these things through intellectual perception. Nevertheless, efficacious union is not effected without knowledge; yet knowledge does not possess a sameness with this union". This is quite opposite to the teaching of the later Hindu writers on Yoga, who make Yoga to consist in knowledge, and also contradicts the implication of what has just been quoted from Lenorment that the efficient means of attaining assimilation with Egyptian divinities was "the knowledge of divine things", unless it mean knowing how to practice Yoga. This efficacious union once attained, the adept may be supposed to perform magical works in the same way as gods do, whatever that may be. But the mode of union is not always the same. Jamblichus says concerning it: "For either divinity possesses us, or we give ourselves wholly to divinity, or we have a common energy with him. And sometimes, indeed, we participate of the last power of divinity, sometimes of his middle, and sometimes of his first power. Sometimes, also, there is participation only, at other times communion likewise, and sometimes a union of these. Again, either the soul alone enjoys the inspiration, or the soul receives it in conjunction with the body, or it is also participated by the common animal " (formed by union of soul and body).

The presence of the invoked deity " is indicated by the motions of the body, and of certain parts of it, by the perfect rest of the body, by harmonious orders and dances, and by elegant sounds, or the contraries of these. Either the body likewise is seen to be elevated, or increased in bulk, or to be borne along sublimely in the air, or the contraries of these are seen to take place about it. An equability, also of voice, according to magnitude, or a great variety of voice after intervals of silence, may be observed. And, again, sometimes the sounds have a musical intension and remission, and sometimes they are strained and relaxed after a different manner".

He who drew down a god saw a spirit descend and enter into some person, and that person was controlled by it. And a species of fire was seen by the recipient, and sometimes by the spectators also, either when the divinity was descended, or when he was departing, from scientifical observation of which what were the powers of the God could be known, and also what he knew and could truly tell. Another indication of the presence of a god was the stupefaction of the person possessed by him, "his own proper consciousness and motion being entirely exterminated", as expressed by Jamblichus, who thence derives an argument for the exclusive agency of the gods, which his queerist had doubted.

First in order among the fruits of Egyptian Yoga was the power of invocation, whereby the gods might be called down and compelled to put themselves in evidence before the multitude, so that none should doubt, and to do and reveal what should be required of them; but this only in a phantasmal way, the gods themselves remaining in heaven the while.

Not only gods, but all beings of "more excellent natures" than men, were thus amenable to theurgic science. Jamblichus devotes ten pages to describing the different orders of these and the signs by which each might be known. Answering the question of Porphery: "By what indication the presence of a god, or an angel, or an archangel, or a daemon, or a certain archon, or a soul, may be known ? " he begins his reply by saying that "their appearance accords with their essences, powers and energies. For such as they are, such also do they appear to those that invoke them, and they exhibit energies and ideas consentaneous to themselves and proper indications of themselves. But that we may descend to particulars, the phantasma or luminous appearances of the gods are uniform; those of daemons are various; those of angels are more simple than those of daemons, but are subordinate to those of the gods; those of archangels approximate in a greater degree to divine; but those of archons (spirits of the planets) will be various", and those of souls will appear to be all various. And the phantasmata, indeed, of the gods will be seen shining with a salutary light; those of archangels will be terrible and at the same time mild; those of daemons will be dreadful; those of heroes are milder than those of daemons ; but those of archons, if their dominion pertains to the world, produce astonishment, but if they are material they are obnoxious and painful to the spectators; and those of souls are similar to the heroic phantasma, except that they are inferior to them". Elsewhere images of souls are said to appear to be "of a shadowy form", The souls thus named as holding the lowest place in the chain of intermediaries were "undefiled souls", who had never incarnated, but had left their companions in heaven to descend among men as ministers of good.

In like manner Jamblichus then goes on to describe each order of intermediaries with respect to essence, energy, movement, attendant retinue, array, accompanying lights and fires, modes of self-purifications, effects produced on men by its presence, tenuity and subtlety of emitted light, and, lastly, influence of the dispositions of the souls of those who evoke them. Other fruits of Egyptian Yoga were: divination of the divine sort, by which the gods are induced to impart such knowledge as they alone possess, which they do by means of dreams, trance-speaking oracles, seeing in water, "eduction of light," meaning the observation of the mutations of light and shadow, and in other ways, thus revealing past and future events and all the secrets of nature; ability to go to inaccessible places ; to float on water ; to move through the air; insensibility to pain; invulnerability to all violence, whether from the hand of man or the physical powers of nature ; superiority over those powers ; immunity from evil spirits and malefic magic; power to make evil and impure souls pure and virtuous; to call down fire from heaven and make statues laugh.

Egyptian sacerdotal magic was practiced as well for the purpose of indirectly controlling the people through the wonders it exhibited and the benefits it conferred, as for obtaining a direct control of their wills of the mesmeric sort, whereby they would be made to do the bidding of their priestly rulers without regard to fear or gratitude, but as of necessity; just as in old Taoism. But no more than the yoga practicers of ancient China did those of ancient Egypt expect deliverance from re-birth to come in the shape of absorption in any god. If Jamblichus speaks of the ascent of the soul after becoming liberated from the bonds of necessity and fate, it is to reinhabit its original home wherein from eternity it had enjoyed its individuality of being; and when he mentions union with a god, he does not mean the god, but such one of the secondary divinities as is specially adapted to do the business in hand, and the union is but for a temporary purpose. And the power thus obtained was not omnipotence nor the knowledge omniscience, the assertions of Jamblichus, which look the other way, to the contrary notwithstanding. But it is easy to see how the lower idea of theurgic union, which certainly prevailed in Egypt to the exclusion of any other, might give birth to the higher one of the Neoplatonists and the still higher one of the Hindus.

Besides sacerdotal theurgy, always considered a branch of magic, magic of a secular sort was largely practiced in Egypt. Practicers of this are probably meant by Jamblichus when he says: " There are a certain few who, by employing a certain supernatural power of intellect, become superior to physical powers". It is probable that this secular magic is the kind referred to in the " Metamorphosis " of Apuleius, that could turn rapid rivers to flow back to their fountains, congeal the sea, take away the Strength of the winds, hold back the sun from his courses, force the moon to scatter her foam, tear the stars from their orbits, take away the day and detain the night. Allusions are also made to magic of much darker hue, in which evil spirits are concerned, which class of beings seem to have performed for Egyptian ecclesiasticism the same kindly office which the Christian devil does for the Christian Church, that of taking the blame for all that goes wrong, and especially for whatever miracle does not testify in that Church's favor.

Concerning the yoga practice of the Egyptian priesthood, whereby its members became prophets, Jamblichus gives hardly a hint. But yoga attainment presupposes quietude and concentration, and that these were Egyptian methods other authorities reveal. He dwells, however, on the magical work by means of which the theurgist once qualified brought himself for the time being into a state of union with a god, or, as it seemed to him, brought the god down to him; these means consisted in temple ritual, and that may be summed up in sacrifice incantation and prayer. Jamblichus defends the sacrificing of animals with a finesse of argument that makes it hard to recognize in the practice our old acquaintance ghostfeeding. Prayer was of three kinds, one of which procured illumination, one communion of operation with the gods, and the third "a perfect plenitude of divine fire". The continual exercise of prayer was supposed to strengthen the intellect, and render the soul receptive to the communications of the gods. Sometimes it was effective without sacrifice, though sacrifice was never effective without it, which allows a suspicion to arise that it was prayer alone — or the concentration of mind involved in it — that did the work, and that the roasted meats really served no other purpose than to replenish the larders of the priests. In their invocations these often used violent language, threatening to raze the temples to the ground, burst the dome of heaven and make known to the world the secrets of Great Isis. Which Jamblichus excuses on the ground that it was in his capacity as temporary god that the priest thus threatened his fellow divinities; and he undertakes also to justify the erection of Phalli and the use of obscene language.

CHAPTER XX - AKKADIAN YOGA

In very early times a portion of the Tauranian race inhabited the mountainous region about the headwaters of the Tigris and Euphrates, named from their habitat Akkadians, or mountaineers, while another portion of the same race dwelt in the neighboring valleys and were known as Sumirians, or lowlanders. In still very early times both moved southward into the lower basin of those rivers, afterwards to be known as Babylonia and Assyria, of which country they were in full possession when the Semites came there, as also of Media, when the Persians conquered it. These Akkadians were a masterful people. Their civilization was certainly as ancient as any we know of. Their system of magic was older than that of Egypt. They invented the cuneiform writing which, inscribed on tiles now being exhumed by tens of thousands, is conveying to the modern world their long-buried history. They, and not Chaldean shepherds, discovered astrology — that is to say, astronomy. A tribe of them, the Kaldu or Kaldi, gave name to all Chaldea, besides dictating to it their magic and religion, while another tribe, the Magii, constituted itself an hereditary priesthood, which at one time became civil rulers also of the Persian Empire. Their criminal laws were mild, and it is most noteworthy that their civil laws accorded to woman large rights, both of person and property, and over her children power above that of the father. Maspero says that the graves and tombs of Chaldea show that a portion of its population burnt the bodies of the dead, and infers that they were the Sumirians, that is, Akkadians, who are by other authorities alleged to have corrupted the religion of the Persians by introducing cremation among them, and to have been the originators of it, in fact. In the refined and spiritual dispositions thus evinced, those of us who do not take our ideas of mortuary decencies from the gravedwellers of Egypt and Chaldea will find another proof of racial superiority. It is also recorded of them that they were able courtiers, which means that they were accomplished gentlemen. Of the branch of them that settled in Finland we learn that their worship was all done in the family, with only the parents for ministers, and that, though they had magicians, they had no priests. Self-reliance that can dispense with priestly aid, though it may imperil souls, must be admitted to be evidence of strong minds and robust wills even in these days, but in times when the aspects and activities of nature were but little understood, and in a region where these were so wonderful and terrible as in Finland, it was surely as heroic a quality as a people could possess. Then as to their literature, the Kalevala is well worthy of a place among the great epic poems of the world.

But the Akkadians, like the Hindus cradled in a robust climate, and, like them, tempted southward into a luxurious but enervating one, found in their new home even a surer, if not more rapid, deterioration than they. Merged in the inferior race they had instructed and civilized, they long ago lost place in history; their language ceased to be spoken three thousand years ago even in countries where it remained a classic and sacred tongue a thousand years longer. And what was the Yoga of this people, so intelligent, receptive and constructive, and of origin so early that their interpretation of the "mystical phenomena of human nature" had the advantage of being first impressions, and their elaboration of them that of untramelled mental freedom? It was neither absorption in a primary god, like that of the Hindus, nor yet assimilation with a secondary one, like that of the Egyptians, but consisted in union of the outerman with an inward entity which yet could not be designated as soul. The Persians names such Fravishis and their descendants, the Parsees, now call them Fervors. Lenorment says, concerning them: "They were the simple essence of all things, the celestial creatures corresponding to the terrestrial, of which they were the immortal types. Every created being had his Fravishi, who was invoked in prayers and sacrifices (the Japanese of to-day prays directly to his ' Lord Soul '), and was the invisible protector, who watched untiringly over the being to whom he was attached". These Fravishis, the same author says, were obviously the Chaldean personal spirits of each being and each object in nature, and that the Chaldeans got the belief in them from the Akkadians, the Finnic branch of which race had the same. He goes on to say: "In the same way that every man had his Fravishi, according to the most recent books of the Avesta, so, also, according to the Akkadian magical tablets — and this doctrine was continually brought out in them — had every man from the hour of his birth a special god attached to him, who lived with him as his protector and as his spiritual type, or, as they expressed the same idea, a divine couple, a god and a goddess, pure spirits". But this god, called so by courtesy, was " of a peculiar character, partaking of human nature its imperfections and foibles". Nor was he as good and powerful as a real god should be. In fact, both the Akkadian cylinders and the Mazdean books make him a part of the soul of his man, though the books spiritualize and make him more perfect than the cylinders do.

But from the well-preserved literature of the Finns, who held on to their old religion and magic until sometime during the middle ages, much more satisfactory information bearing on this subject can be obtained. Says M. Lenorment: "According to the Finnish creed, each man bore within him from his birth a divine spirit who was his inseparable companion for life. The spirit became more closely united to its subject in proportion as the latter tore himself away from earthly things to enter into the sanctuary of his soul. This was an important source of the magician's supernatural power; he aspired to a transcendental ecstasy, tiilla-tntoon, to a great state of excitement of the soul, tulla haltiorhiri in which he became like the spirit dwelling in him, and entirely identified with it. He used artificial means, intoxicating drugs for instance, in order to attain to this state of excitement, for it was only then, so to speak, that he succeeded in deifying himself. This doctrine, which M. Rien has explained very clearly, and which held a chief place in the Finnish religious ideas, as also in their magic, is just that of the special god attached to each man and dwelling in his body, which prevailed also in the Akkadian magical books. This furnishes an affinity of conceptions and beliefs which is of great importance, since it is not one of those natural ideas which arise independently among widely different nations. To find elsewhere a similar notion, we must go to Persia for the doctrines of the Fravishis. " But if it is not " one of those natural ideas which arise independently among different nations, "the natural phenomena upon which it rests are precisely what do so arise, for they depend on what is inherent in human nature; and these being given, the ideas will come of themselves, with such general similarity and special variation as may be expected of the workings of the same human mind in varying conditions of time, place and circumstance. From the above we see that Akkadian Yoga consisted in an union; was accompanied by an ecstasy, a trance; was best attainable through renunciation of earthly thmgs and seclusion ; was aided by intoxicating drugs, like the soma of the Hindus, and invested the successful practicer with magical powers. Concentration of mind, though implied in the foregoing, is not directly named in the authorities consulted; but whoso will look through the tens of thousands of tiles now being exhumed, will hardly fail to find the word concentration there. The Akkadian magicians performed their work as such, as also did their gods, almost wholly by incantation. Their Finnic representatives according to the Kalevala did the same, Wainamoinen, "ancient bard and famous singer":

" Sang aloft a famous pine-tree, " Till it pierced the clouds in growing " With its golden top and branches, " Till it touched the very heavens. " Now he sings again enchanting, " Sings the moon to shine forever " In the fir-tree's emerald branches, " In the top he sings the Great Bear".

Another singer, Lemminkainen :

" Quick began his incantations, " Straightway sang the songs of witchcraft: " From his fur robe darts the lightning. " Flames outshooting from his eye-balls, " From the magic of his singing, " From his wonderful enchantment, " Sang the very best of singers " To (be) the very worst of minstrels, " Filled their mouths with dust and ashes, " Piled the rocks upon their shoulders, " Stilled the best of Lapland witches, " Stilled the sorcerers and witches".

Nor did he stop until he had either bewitched or banished all save one within the sound of his voice. And just as the human magicians did, Ukko, the creative divinity of the Finns, worked chiefly by incantation. He could " Sing the origin of matter, " Sing the legends of omniscience, " Sing his songs in full perfection. " God could sing the floods to honey, " Sing the sands to ruddy berries, " Sing the pebbles into barley. " Sing to beer the running waters, " Sing to salt the rocks of ocean, " Into cornfields sing the forests, " Into gold the forest fruitage, " He could touch the springs of magic", etc. " He could turn the keys of nature", etc.

And even Finnic small birds sang into existence the trees whose branches they perched on.

CHAPTER XXI - MOHAMMEDAN YOGA

Like every other revealed religion, Mohammedanism had magic for its root; but it was poor in quality and scant in quantity. Its founder was, like every other founder, a practicer of yoga, but he was a very partially developed one, notwithstanding his frequent retreats within the grotto of Mount Hera, where, during twenty years of his life, he was accustomed to receive communications by the mouth of Gabriel. As a man, so ignorant that it is doubted if he could read or write, as a saint he never attained to that stage in the path where intuition comes in to supply the want of learning. He had reached the stage of "meditation", but not that of "spiritual contemplation", as John of the Cross called the one which lies next beyond ; nor had he gone very far in meditation either, which is the state wherein, as the same saint tells us, voices are heard and visions seen and by other exterior methods the mind is addressed through the senses, for he could not boast of having seen the angel in his real form more than twice, whereas Swedenborg claimed to have seen and conversed with Jesus Christ himself "thousands of times". He had not even attained to the power of working miracles wherewith to set the seal to his revelations, unless the pure style of Arabic in which they were clothed may be considered such, as, in fact, he claimed it to be. The Koran is by reason of its diffuseness and repetitions made to cover some five hundred pages, though its solid contents could easily have been compressed into ten. Its language is often rugged and commonplace, as befits a discourse by an ignorant man to ignorant men, like that of Joe Smith, the Mormon prophet or, an untaught Methodist exhorter; and though one versed in Arabic might find its double-rhymed lines agreeable to the ear, he not so versed, who attempts to read it in English, is apt to lay it down before the end is reached as the most tiresome book he ever took up. It is made up mostly of threats of eternal punishment violently and with much ranting denounced against whoever will not take Mohammed's word for it that Allah is the one only God and he his latest prophet. Now, in this Allah, though at the time acting as chief of all other Arabian gods, and therefore often styled, like the Jehovah of the Jews, Most High, we recognize our former acquaintance who jointly with his wife the terrible Allat ruled over the Chaldean hell ; so it is not wonderful that threats are more to his mind than persuasion, or that instead of employing a rival deity to do the punishing, as is usual, he attends to it personally. For every page of the Koran there is a threat that he will "torment " disbelieving or disobeying sinners, and throughout it such expressions abound as — "I will broil you in hell fire" — " I will pour boiling water over you" — "I will make you to drink boiling water". But with all these are mingled oft-repeated assurances that his pity and mercy are unbounded, for every sin but unbelief, that is to say he will pardon all offenders against others than himself ; which must needs greatly weaken the effect of his fulminations, since they threaten, in effect to send to hell only those who don't believe he can do it. Accordingly, his prophet had in the end to adopt the method of cutting off heads after the manner of King Clovis in evangelizing the Saxons, and with like good results. Thus, except that Mohammed's few first conversions, mostly of relatives and friends who may be presumed to have believed him when he related his experiences in the grotto, Mohammedanism owes little or nothing to magic. Favoring circumstances, burning zeal and good politics acting in aid of the sword must have their share of credit. Then the simplicity of the new religion is to be considered. No priest, no authority, Allah, Mohammed and the last day for creed. Circumcision for the only sacrament, five easy ablutions and as many short prayers daily for ritual, and the golden rule for moral law, are not hard to understand nor very hard to conform to. Equally simple are the methods of punishment and reward ; roasting forever in hell or living forever in a paradise where crystal fountains are eternal in play and bowers of roses eternal in bloom, whereon loll and languish beautiful virgins eternal in bud.

Such was the simple cult that raised to whatever elevation they have attained a race of low-minded, drunken, licentious and cruel robbers and murderers.

Though at the start without any such magical, that is, miraculous, support as Christianity had in the works of Jesus and his disciples, Mohammedanism after it had taken form and got upon its legs could not have lacked such attestations, for no religion has. Among a body of earnest devotees, such as newly made converts ever are, there will always be found some of mediumistic natures to whom, through devotional concentration, devotional ecstasy will come, either as the " inner witness " of intuition or the outer one of visions and voices, always testifying according to the preconceptions of receivers, to keep alive the lamp of faith and fire of zeal in themselves and kindle them in others. But when the movement spread to more enlightened countries, such as Chaldea and Persia, where the old magic of Akkadia had for thousands of years prevailed, it could not have been long in drawing to its support yoga adepts of superior sort, able to exhibit the usual signs and wonders which are supposed to infallibly attest religious truth. Such are the Sufis and others, systematic practicers of yoga under true yoga conditions, selfrenouncing ascetics, associated in communities each of which, so independent are they of all authority in respect to belief or discipline, constitutes a sect by itself, while most of them must be considered as quite apart from the Mohammedanism the

Prophet taught. These, notwithstanding their heretical character, hold Islam together in a solidarity such as neither the Koran nor the Sonna could be deemed adequate to effect, supplying a soul to the body which the creed, ritual and law constitute. In their teachings are included heresies like these: There is one truth for the wise which is absolute, and another for the ignorant which is relative — absolute pantheism — direct communion with heaven obtainable by austerities — there is no free-will, God being the All-doer as well as the Allmighty — the stories of heaven and hell are mere allegories — reason only leads to error; intuition alone is infallible. To reconcile such doctrines as these with the Koran its obvious sense is either flatly contradicted or cruelly wrenched; and it is not to be wondered at that the "officiants and savants" of Islamism, as a French writer says, accuse the teachers of them of heterodoxy. Nevertheless, the religious orders, by their pure and disinterested lives, have won and largely enjoy the respect and attachment of the people.

Of the Sufis M. Lemairesse says: "The mystic Sufi becomes absorbed in his contemplation and love. Four degrees conduct him to assimilation with God".

"The first is humanity, or the ordinary life of mankind, in which he is given up wholly to his passions".

" The second degree, or the path, is properly the doctrinal initiation; the initiate who comprehends God is released from devotional observances".

" The third degree is knowledge".

" The trials which have to be endured in attaining to this degree are so severe that often the subject succumbs ; if he succeeds in overcoming them, he becomes the equal of the angels, his spirit comes into possession of the faculty which forms its essence, intuition of the true nature of beings, perception of all things from the throne of God down to the rain-drop".

" The fourth degree is beatitude, and is obtained by a fast nearly absolute of forty days; after it the disciple goes into the desert where he abstains from all manual occupation and has no communication with any one but his director. The ordeal accomplished, the ascetic participates in the divine nature and has the power to work miracles".

But the order of the Kheloutya make the progress towards perfection consist of seven degrees instead of four, which are as follows:

" In the first degree, that of humanity, he perceives ten thousand lights, dull and intermixed, and he can see genii".

" In the second, that of passionate ecstasy, he perceives, besides, ten thousand blue lights".

" The third degree is the ecstasy of the heart. He sees hell and its attributes, also the genii and all theirs".

" The fourth degree is the ecstasy of the immaterial soul. He sees ten thousand new lights of bright yellow; also souls of prophets and saints".

" The fifth degree is the mysterious ecstasy. Here he sees the angels and ten thousand lights more, of brilliant white".

" In the sixth degree, that of the ecstasy of obsession, he sees ten thousand other lights, as of a limpid mirror, feels a delicious spiritual ravishment, and beholds the prophets".

"At length he arrives at the seventh degree, that of beatitude; then appear ten thousand more lights, green and white, but which undergo successive transformations until they light up to view the attributes of God and certain words of the Lord recorded in the Sonna are heard. He seems no longer to belong to this world, all terrestrial things disappear".

After these two prominent examples of Mohammedan Yoga in which are found: contemplation; absorption in God ; release from devotional observances ; intuitive knowledge of the nature of all beings; bliss; power to work miracles; the joytis or lights in connection with the five tatwic colors (assuming to be red the one mistaken for hell-fire) ; there is hardly needed to completely prove the kinship of this with other systems, the following incidents and requirements gleaned from the " conclusion " written at the end of his translation of "the Rauzat-us-Safa" by M. Lemairesse concerning the religious orders of Islam: seclusion; solitude; silence; abstinence ; fasts ; vigils ; non-attachment ; renunciation ; poverty ; much repetition of formulas, especially of the sacred word Allah, Yoga relates to the entire man, therefore its literature cannot ignore his love. Thus, having passed in review the Hindu mudras and the Chinese story of Nii Yii, we now come to what the great Thaumaturge Mahmed ben Aissa has to say in his instructions to the order he founded concerning one kind of love: "Mysterious or secret love consists in absorbing one's self completely in God. When he has arrived at communication with the interior love of God, duality becomes unity. Luminous spirits are seen. One loses the sense of self and of modesty; one is wholly filled with the breath of divinity". To which words of mystery the remark of the translator, that "probably there are special and, above all, eccentric details reserved for adepts further advanced in initiation", seem quite appropriate. Thus, after the proselyting sword of Islam had swept over the territory where Akkadian magic aud the religion allied to it had so long flourished, leveling in its course both religion and magic, there sprouted from the stubble a new form of magic, to seize upon and modify the new religion as the old had the old ones; a new form, but of an old thing. For Mohammedan Yoga is yoga still. Just how far association with Mohammedanism has altered its appearance, how far a more modern philosophy has re-formulated it, how far experience has improved its methods, how far it is unitary and how far fragmentary, we are hindered from knowing by the circumstances that the religious orders, for their protection against the criticism of orthodoxy, are become secret orders as well. But this much is known, that, profiting by the large freedom within the fold allowed to his flock by the Prophet, the members of them indulge in a variety of doctrine and practice both of yoga and religion such as no Christian church has ever tolerated within its pale — though had all Christian churches done so they might have saved themselves a deal of trouble and the world a deal of misery. And the better support afforded to Mohammedanism by its contemplative communities as compared with that which Christianity gets from those which it permits but severely regulates, testifies that if the Church had allowed more freedom it would have got in return more strength.

CHAPTER XXII - HEBREW YOGA

According to the history of the Jews, as written by themselves, they were truly a peculiar people, and their Jehovah a peculiar god. They seem to have never tired of sinning in his sight nor he of punishing them for it. Within the three hundred years from Joshua to Saul he had to discipline them by delivering them into the hands of their mutual enemies, to endure terms of slavery varying from eight to eighteen years, no less than six several times; nor in all these centuries is any one good action recorded of him. His terrible judgments were almost exclusively visited on offenders against himself, or if he did now and then undertake to render justice between man and man, it was the wrong man that got punished. A brutal race prone to carnage and destruction he was continually commanding to kill and burn, or punishing for slackness in doing so. And the wonder is equal that of all the nations of the earth any god should have chosen such a people for his own, and that of all the hosts of heaven any people should have chosen such a god.

To understand why he so often and severely punished them for "sinning in his sight", it must be considered that the sinning in question consisted in worshiping other gods, which in turn consisted in roasting on their altars the rams and bullocks he coveted for his own, and that inasmuch as in those days gods needed food and drink as well as other people, service of god meant table-service, and the worship of Baal by the Jews meant the starvation of Jehovah. The cause of this incorrigible disposition to backslide evidently was that the worship of the gods of the surrounding nations was more attractive to the Jews than their own. All those nations were the disciples of the Egyptians and Akkadians, especially of the latter, and had a splendid ritual and potent theurgy that irresistibly allured to their temples the ignorant, uns-table flock whom Moses had tried to indoctrinate in his newly. formulated faith. High adept as he was, he could not control them, though he proved his ability to prophesy when, just before he died, he foretold that no one else would ever be able to do so.

"And there arose not a prophet since in Israel like unto Moses, whom the Lord knew face to face", His successors, the judges, enjoyed no such advantage as he had while a student of magic under the learned Egyptian priests. The judges were not celibates, nor given to contemplation. What mystical faculty they had must have come, as modern mediumship does, suddenly, with out discipline, only occasionally amounting to "open vision". In Samuel's time there was none at all; "and the word of the Lord was precious (rare) in those days; there was no open vision". Down to the time of Elijah and Elisha the " signs " they exhibited as warrant for their claims to authority were few and insignificant. Samuel relied on his prediction of a thunder shower to attest his. " So Samuel called unto the Lord and the Lord sent thunder and rain that day: and all the people greatly feared the Lord and Samuel". A prophet was not educated, he was " raised up" ,or, " The Spirit of the Lord came upon him". Like a nervous disease, the faculty of foresight was infectious : " And when they saw the company of the prophets prophesying, and Samuel standing as appointed over them, the Spirit of God was on the messengers of Saul, and they too prophesied. " Others sent were seized by the same spirit, and again others, and finally when the King went himself, he was attacked by it so strongly that he stripped off his clothes (as insane people sometimes do) and prophesied before Samuel in like manner, "and lay down naked all that day and all that night". But though the suddenness of their development and their limited powers indicate that the sages raised up to rule and judge Israel during the centuries of theocratic government were not advanced beyond a very rudimentary stage, yet, when later, with the establishment of monarchical government, the social state of the tribes became so far ameliorated as to permit of ascetic seclusion to candidates for adeptship, which was about two centuries after Samuel, prophets of a very high order appeared. The first was Elijah the Thisbite, "a hairy man, wearing a girdle of leather about his loins". Confident in his power, even to arrogance, he declared to King Ahab : "As the Lord God of Israel liveth before whom I stand, there shall not be dew nor rain these years, but according to my word". Then, going into hiding, probably to avoid punishment for his arrogance, he was fed by ravens. Afterwards to repay a widow for her hospitality he made her scant store of food inexhaustible, and later restored her dead son to life. Next, he challenged all the prophets of Baal to a contest of magical skill, the test being the calling down of fire from heaven to consume the offering on the altar, and, having triumphed, killed them one and all. King Ahaziah sent a captain of fifty with his fifty to summon him into his presence, but he promptly killed them with fire from heaven ; likewise a second captain with his fifty sent on the same errand ; and a third detachment only escaped by humble supplication for mercy ; then he went to the King and boldly condemned him to death for having sent messengers to Baal-ze-bub, the God of Ekron, to enquire if he should recover his health. For his latest miracle Elijah smote with his mantle the waters of Jordan, so that he and his pupil Elisha crossed over on dry land. Finally, and after imparting to Elisha a double portion of his spirit, he stepped into a chariot of fire with horses of fire, and was carried up by a whirlwind into Heaven.

Elisha, taking up the mantle that fell from his master as he ascended, begun the exercise of magical power now first developed in him after some ten years of teaching, by performing with it a like miraculous parting of waters. After which his miracles were the following: — He purified poisonous waters — called out of the woods two bears to kill forty-two children for jeering at his tonsure — after refreshing his power by listening to music, made a valley-full of water issue from the earth — from a single pot of oil filled an indefinite number of others — gave a son to a woman having an aged husband — restored that son to life when completely dead — made healthy food of a pottage of poisonous herbs — with twenty loaves of barley and full ears of corn fed an hundred men — healed one leper and made another — caused an axe of iron to float in water — informed his King that his enemy the King of Syria was plotting against him in the privacy of his far-distant chamber — called to his aid against a host sent to capture him a mountain ful of chariots and horses of fire — smote the same host with blindness — And even after his death his bones restored to life another dead man who was touched by them.

Here were adepts indeed ! and such as are not made in a day. Assuming to be true the accounts given of them by historians who stood in the same relation to them and their works that the four evangelists did to Jesus and his, both Elijah and Elisha, though bad enough to be fit intermediaries between the Jews of those days and their God, were as great prophets as any that are named in Jewish or Christian records, not excepting even Jesus of Nazareth. Both of them healed the sick, raised the dead, caused scanty portions of food to fill many mouths and made the waters obey them; while either one or the other of them (or both) could call down from heaven fire or water at discretion, or blight the earth with drought terminable only at his will — could render poisoned pottage safe to eat and poisoned springs safe to drink from, fill with water dry ditches, compel wild birds to bring him food or wild beasts to execute his vengeance, confer offspring upon senile impotence, or hear words privately spoken in a distant city. What their methods were for attaining to such power no record tells, but Akkadian magic was practiced in all the countries around them, and we may be sure that the Jews received and practiced it as early as they became civilized enough to do so. As no prophets came after the above two that could be said to excel them, none others need be noticed until we come to Jesus of Nazareth.

Jesus of Nazareth

The historical portions of the Old Testament, allowance being made for a patriotic disposition on the part of the writers of it to magnify the exploits of the Jewish armies, especially in relation to the numbers of their enemies killed in battle or slaughtered afterwards, may be taken to be reasonably well founded in fact. The narrative of the earlier books was written by men too ignorant to plagiarize and too unimaginative to invent, and in a simple truth-like style. Down to the time of the Kings the statements of so-called supernatural occurrences are so moderate as to be matched and more than matched by the accounts now current and largely credited of like occurrences in our own day. This being so in the earlier parts, where error and falsity would be most apt to get in, the presumption in favor of the later ones is thereby strengthened. Except that Moses was believed to have spoken with Jehovah face to face, and that Elijah claimed to "stand before" him, the modes of revelation by which the Jews supposed the word of God was conveyed to them were of no higher order than our modern spiritual communications. They consisted in dreams, visions, trance speaking, speaking by impression, automatic writing, direct writing, clairvoyance, clairaudience, drawing lots, and the temple oracle, supposed to have been chrystal-seeing. The Hebrew bible does not claim to be the word of God in any other sense than as recording these. It should be judged by its own claim rather than those set up for it by a Christian council, and thus judged must be decided to be a rasonably credible history, as sacred histories go.

But for many reasons no such credit can be accorded to the New Testament, which is obviously so distorted and encumbered by priestly and controversial tampering, to say nothing of the honest errors of ignorance, that in general it would not be worth one's while to attempt to straighten out or disencumber it ; certainly not worth the while of one able to see that it may be admitted to be true in every part without at all proving any one of the hundreds of creeds, heretical or orthodox, that men have attempted to build upon it — because able to see nothing more in it than the story of a great yogi who some nineteen hundred years ago in Palestine "went about doing good". Yet it is well at the outset of our enquiry to get rid of the objection often made, that since the silence of contemporaneous history concerning Herod's massacre of the innocents and the prodigies connected with the birth and death of Jesus, all claimed to have happened in times when every important event was carefully verified, reported and put on record by the Roman officials, disproves the accounts of them contained in the gospels, that silence, therefore, disproves the gospels themselves, with their whole content. But there is no vital connection between the statements in question and the rest of the story, from which they may easily be detached. The fable of the massacre may be dismissed as an old one, told once against Nimrod and again against Pharaoh, besides others; while as to the prodigies, is it not known that down to the times in question it was usual to put them in as preface and appendix to biographies of great religious leaders, to give to one of whom a celestial phenomenon for a harbinger and an earthquake for a funeral was nothing more than historical courtesy required ? Even distinguished civil rulers were often complimented in the same way — Julius Caesar, for instance, and the Emperors Augustus, Claudius, Nero and Vespasian.

But there are in the gospels two statements, specifically affirmed and insisted on, relating to the advent and departure of their subject, that, if true, make him a god and not a yogi. And these are not to be summarily disposed of, for both have a plausible groundwork in magical and, therefore, natural phenomena. The one relates to the divine paternity, and the other to the resurrection, neither of which, I think, has a counterpart in any other religion, for though pagan gods habitually become fathers of men, they never incarnated in their sons, and though they habitually dwelt in heaven, none of them had to die on earth in order to get there. But the phenomena in question will account for both the older and simpler interpretation and the newer and more complex one, while their true meaning will be found, at the least, as momentous as either. A resurrection of the body is something capable of proof or disproof; not so a divine paternity or incarnation of god or man. But there are facts in nature which account for the beliefs which have obtained in all of these, and so deprive them of any power to prove themselves true by the mere fact of their having got into men's minds.

In his "Philosophy of Mysticism" Baron Du Prel treats of a "curative instinct of nature", which continually acts by the various modes of communication possible between the occult and the manifest self of man, to influence the latter for its own preservation, which modes are many and various, ranging from vague impressions of impending evil and the cravings of pregnancy up to objectified visions of celestial messengers, warning against disaster, and are adapted to the receptivities of those sought to be influenced by them. Now, the sexual faculty lies quite within the sphere of this curative instinct; in fact, according to Hindu science, the organs of that faculty are the seat of all occult power, the power that operates the signals. When an ascetic devotee in his cave or cell has by those very pious concentrations practiced to keep down desire, roused it up, and the vision of a beautiful woman arises, whom he takes for the devil and commands to avaunt, maybe it is not the devil at all that is tempting him, but his own soul, that he is wearing out his miserable body in efforts to save, that is trying to tell him what would be good to take to preserve that body. A relieving orgasm is commonly brought on by a dream, as is well known, but it is claimed that sometimes, dreams failing. Nature, who, as Schopenhauer says, will not be frustrated if she can help it, goes so far as to call up, or project rather, an apparition that is present to the waking eye, or to both sight and touch, or to touch without sight, or to all the senses. Here are suggested the old persistent tales of incubi and succubi, of Count Galbas and his sub-mundanes, and stories whispered of experiences now going on in this country, some of which it is even asserted have tested and proved the possibility of bodily touch projected from a distant body, of a kind that suggests Jupiter's visits to Psyche. According to Swami Swatmaram, a man who has become proficient in the difficult Vagroli Mudra has power to attract to himself "the damsels of the Siddhas"; and a woman properly developed by intercourse with him becomes a yogini, and among other miraculous gifts has that of being able to "go through the air " to somebody, just as at the call of Krishna from the woods those of his 12,000 milkmaid wives, whose earthly husbands held them back, sent their souls, and got to the god before those others could who went on foot. We have seen that one of the Mohammedan religious orders has a book of instructions in which "mysterious or secret love" is mentioned as belonging to a very advanced state of ecstasy wherein " spirits of light appear", and one loses the feeling of self and of modesty"; " one is filled with the breath of God". Saint John of the Cross, the Christian ascetic, has left behind him some verses describing the loves of the soul and its bridegroom Jesus, of which a few here quoted will show the tendency of one kind of love to run into another, under certain conditions:

" In the dark night, " With anxious love inflamed, " O, happy lot! " Forth, unobserved I went, " My house being now at rest. " In darkness and in safety, " By the secret ladder, disguised, " O, happy lot!

" In darkness and concealment, " My house being now at rest.

*****

" There he gave me his breasts, " There he taught me the science full of sweetness, "And there I gave to him, " Myself without reserve, " There I promised to be his bride".

But inasmuch as a truly virtuous woman would never, dreaming or awake, receive another than her husband, to obtain access to such an one a god must come, or seem to come, and thus a belief that the visitor is a divine one arises from the nature of the case; how from a mere objectified illusion so substantial a thing as a male child could result is another question. We know that by manual operation the human germ has been deposited in the matrix and there fecundated. Many careful observers of our spiritual phenomena believe that far more bulky and ponderable objects than that germ can be by some occult means moved from place to place, passing through material obstructions on the way, or materialize on the spot. Perhaps the most reasonable hypothesis yet suggested to account for such phenomena is that the subconscious self of some living person present is the agent. If so, then in every such case of love-making by an objectified illusion, there being neither a real man nor a real god present, the agent is presumably the sub-conscious woman, and the phenomenon may properly be termed self-visitation, to which the next step could only be self-impregnation. Such are the suppositions which, if well founded, reduce an immaculate conception to the rank of an orderly creative process.

Moreover, there were afloat in those times traditional beliefs of magical impregnation. The divine infant of which the Finnic virgin Mariatta was the mother and a wild strawberry the putative father was, according to the Kalevala, at first refused baptism on the ground that it was a child of witchcraft. The same scripture also records another miraculous conception and birth in these words:

"Time had gone but little distance " Ere a boy was born in magic "Of the virgin, Untamala".

*****

" Then they laid the child of wonder, " Fatherless, the magic infant, " In the cradle of attention".

And as late as the time of Jacob Boehme, that visionary in his treatise on "The Way to Christ", wrote that God's first intent when he created Adam was that he should be self-impregnating, and therefore he was made bi-sexual, but that even before he was tested by temptation, happening to foresee that he never could stand it, he gave him a wife, "For God saw that Adam could not then generate magically".

Certainly something must have been going on in the world to give rise to the many stories we have both of magical begettings and of matrons and virgins giving birth to sons of gods. Such are to be found in probably every book of scripture of whatever religion has owned one. Self-visitation and impregnation, if they can be supposed to be possible, would account for them all. The woman, for reasons just given, would in each case feel sure it was none other than a god that came to her, while others, if satisfied there was no access of any man could hardly help agreeing with her. But it is not vital to any thesis of this writing that the above theory should be established, and it is only advanced to show that certain beliefs are not without supporting facts, and as a help to thinkers disposed to inquire into the meaning of the facts.

The story of the Resurrection of Jesus, so much relied on by believers as proving their religion and by disbelievers as, by its absurdity, disproving it, had it been told in India would have caused little astonishment and no skepticism, so used to such things are they there. Says Swatmaram: "Siva, Matsyendra, Sahara, Ananda, Bhairava, Chourangi, Meena, Goraksha, Virupaksha, Bilesa, Manthana, Bhairava, Siddhi, Buddha, Kanthadi, Korantaka, Surananda Siddhapada, Charpati, Kaneri, Pujyapada, Nityanatha, Niranjana, Kapalika, Bindunatha, Kaka, Chandeeswara, Allabha, Prabhudeva, Ghoda, Chodi, Sentmi, Bhanuki, Naradeva, Khanda, Kapalki, and many other great Siddhas, having conquered time, move about the world". They had by pushing yoga practice to the end made themselves perfect yogis, and thus identified with Brahman, but had not as yet departed this life. In Hindu belief such beings can postpone their departure as long as they will, and sometimes do so for thousands of years, meanwhile "moving about the world". Such, too, was the belief of the Taoists of ancient China. Chuang-Tzu declared that when he wrote he was twelve hundred years old, nothing was known of Lao-Tsee's dying at all ; on the contrary, it is recorded that when last seen he was traveling westward just as Finnic Wainamoinen and Schlatter, the wonderful American healer, did when they too disappeared. The Finnic Christ disappeared when he was but an infant. Pythagoras was by some of his disciples believed to have not perished in the burning house, but to have merely passed out of sight. Romulus also was by the Romans thought to have disappeared without dying. Longfellow's "Hiawatha" records a belief held by the North American Indians that their great prophets did so too. The epic " Kalevala " contains the following description of sailing away of the great magician Wainamoinen from his Finland home:

" Sang his farewell song to Northland, " To the people of Wainola, " Sang himself a boat of copper,

"Beautiful his bark of Magic ; " At the helm sat the magician, " Sat the ancient wisdom-singer. " Westward, westward sailed the hero. " Thus the ancient Wainamoinen, " In his copper-banded vessel, " Left his tribe in Kalevala, " Sailing o'er the rolling billows, " Sailing through the azure vapors, " Sailing through the dusk of evening, " Sailing to the fiery sunset, " To the higher landed regions, " To the lower verge of heaven, " Quickly gained the far horizon, " Gained the purple colored harbor, " There his bark he firmly anchored, " Rested in his bark of copper; " But he left his harp of magic, " Left his songs and wisdom-sayings, " To the lasting joy of Suomi".

The poem also hints at the possibility of the subsequent return of the departing sage:

" That I may bring back the Sampo, " Bring anew the harp of joyance, " Bring again, the golden moonlight, " Bring again the silver sunshine, " Peace and plenty to the Northland".

Concerning the anomalous state of being of such departants Chuang-Tzu gives a hint of the old Chinese doctrine, when he says that one who has attained to Tao is "it for translation".

The Hebrew Bible says: "And Enoch lived sixty and five years, and begat Methuselah: and Enoch walked with God after he begat Methuselah three hundred years, and begat sons and daughters; and all the days of Enoch were three hundred and sixty-five years; and Enoch walked with God: and he was not; for God took him". Which seems plainly enough to mean that he was a yogi who after attaining to junction with God lived in the world for three hundred years more and then disappeared, The Mohammedan Rauzat-Us-Safa describes Enoch as being constantly engaged in meditation and prayer, and states that when he was eighty-two years old he managed to get into Paradise and once there refused to leave it. It is noteworthy in this connection that although every other antediluvian from Adam to Noah (except Lamech, who lived to seven hundred and seventy) was allowed more than nine hundred years of life, this companion of God and the only perfected saint of them all was given only three hundred and sixty-five. Why was his stay on earth thus cut short unless that he might be advanced to a better state? It is also noteworthy that during the last three hundred years of his earthly activity he was in two states of" being at once, walking with God in the one and raising a family in the other. These years of earthly activity may be considered as a continuing return.

The Mohammedans also say that Enoch returned to earth as Elijah and the Christians say that Elijah returned to be present at the Transfiguration, where he and Moses were seen talking with Jesus. Was Moses then still alive, having disappeared, not died? It is true that in Deuteronomy it is said that he died, but that was the only account of his disappearance that in those times the ignorant Jews could understand; and some account must be given them. But the next two verses read thus : "And he buried him in a valley in the land of Moab, over against Bethlehem, but no man knoweth of his sepulchre unto this day. And Moses was an hundred and twenty years old when he died: his eye was not dim, nor his natural force abated". Now that a man should bury his own dead body is inconceivable; so it is that one in the prime of life should go and hide himself away, to die in some place that would serve as a tomb. But that a perfected yogi, one "fit for translation" as we are quite at liberty to believe Moses was, healthy and strong, as such are able by their art always to keep themselves, and by the same art able at will to disappear from view or "move about the world"; also able to foreknow the dismal life before him if he continued his hitherto unavailing efforts to make a decent people out of the brutal tribes he had so long "carried in his bosom"; as shown by the prophecy of their future ill-doings which he delivered to them as a farewell address— that such an one should have at last got tired and disgusted and secretly and quietly abandoned them to their wretched fate, is quite conceivable. Supposing it to have been so, there were present at that Transfiguration the only two persons mentioned in Jewish scripture as having, without undergoing death, disappeared from life and subsequently returned, not as re-incarnated souls of the dead, but as the original men. Was yet a third one there present?

What is the mode of being of such after disappearance, what their place, state and activity, has been much speculated upon but never determined, yet this much is certain and could be proved by many other citations than the above, a belief has always existed that the perfected magical adept has the power to take his own time for dying, and meanwhile can come and go in the earth at will.

The different and conflicting accounts we have of the crucifixion of Jesus leave it quite open to belief that he was not dead when taken down from the cross. The time required to kill a man by crucifixion was, according to M. Paul de Regla, often as much as three days, rarelyless than two. But owing to the nearness of the Sabbath Jesus was allowed to hang only three hours, and that without receiving any mortal hurt. The same writer says that in practice the feet were not nailed, that they sometimes touched the ground, being merely tied to the tree by the ankles, and that a projecting block of wood served as a sort of saddle on which the most of the sufferer's weight might rest. Jesus escaped the coup de grace, which consisted in breaking the limbs, by appearing to be dead, though the lance-thrust proved the contrary, for it drew blood, and blood cannot flow from a corpse. The appearance of death may perfectly well have been from a trance, induced by the very intensity of the pain suffered, such as has often happened to those habituated to trance, as all yogis are. Thus it was by some power so ordered that the crucifixion should not kill Jesus of Nazareth — might it not have been his own magical power ? He was certainly magician enough for that, and also to close the eyes of the keepers, walk forth from the sepulchre at the proper time, and give the women the vision of the angels. All this would have been quite consistent with his going voluntarily to his trial and execution.

If, on the above grounds, the gospel story can be considered as rid of hindrances to belief that have been considered valid because not understood, there remains a story that, whether true or false, carries no falsity on its face — of a great magician and good man, exhibiting only fallible wisdom, and no powers higher than Elijah and Elisha manifested when they went about doing evil. I think the foregoing shows that the story of the resurrection is not absurd enough to prove the four gospels untrue, nor yet wonderful enough to prove them true.

CHAPTER XXIII - YOGA OF THE ESSENES

Some two or more centuries B. C. a fanatical order of ascetic Jews established themselves near the western borders of the Dead Sea. They were communists, celibates, diligent in work and devotion, cultivated quietude of body and mind and an humble deportment, wearing their garments to rags, though practicing frequent ablutions, dressed in white and wore long hair, recruited their numbers by adopting young children and also admitting adults tired of the world, and wandering much from city to city, but never begging, A few of the more intelligent among them, by retreat and contemplation, became adepts, and ruled the others with great rigor, giving forth to them teachings of an exoteric kind, while reserving to themselves an esoteric freedom of thought and inspiration. These devoted themselves largely to science and philosophy, and many of them became healers as well as prophets. Whatever the magical attainments of the Essenes were, they gave proof, when subjected to martyrdom, of having acquired the philosophical equanimity in its highest degree, their insensibility to, or disregard of pain being such that they could smile while undergoing the most terrible torture, chat pleasantly with their executioners, and die joyfully. The Therapeuts of Egypt were very much like the Essenes, and the two sects are often confounded with one another in the scant historical accounts we have of them. Some of the Essenes were severely ascetic, and took the name of Nazarenes.

Robert Taylor, in his Diegesis, as well as many other writers, have held the theory that Jesus was an Essene, but against this several objections arise. He always talked and acted as a free man, owing accountability to no authority, whereas the Essenes were strictly disciplined and held under slavish control by their superiors. When arrested and tried, not one friend appeared in his behalf, whereas the Essenes were a large and powerful sect and corporation, more numerous, says M. De Regla, than the Sadducees, and would hardly have let an important confrere be the victim of a farcical trial, wanton ignominy and cruel death. They were not mendicants, but diligent producers and owners of property, and in each city one of their number was ready to supply the wants of travelling members; but no mention is made of the wandering Nazarene having had any such recourse. The Essenes were bigoted Sabbath-keepers; he was a daring Sabbath-breaker. Finally, no mention of the Essenes is made in any of the gospels in which accounts of the Pharisees and Sadducees so abound.

CHAPTER XXIV - THE ROMAN STOICS AS YOGIS

When the Roman people had reached that stage of development in which a craving for philosophy is felt and religion loses its hold on instructed men, there arose the sect of Stoics, which, reacting to the rude and stirring conditions that still prevailed, became in many respects different from any other, both as to doctrine and conduct. The Stoics were not true, contemplative yogis; they were too busy with the active affairs of life for that, yet in their lives and teachings they showed that Akkadian magic and its accompanying philosophy had not in its westward extension stopped at the eastern shores of the Mediterranean. They believed in an universal soul, of which all individual ones are but manifestations, and into which they are destined to be finally absorbed. They believed in the persistence of life after death, and that death only restores man to the state he held before birth, though on both these points their opinions varied and altered, as needs must be when the mind reaches out towards the unknowable. They held the things and affairs of human life in contempt, and if using or enjoying them disregarded them, which is no other than the renunciation and non-attachment of the Hindus. They had no personal god, no future rewards or punishments, hence no fear of death. "Where we are, "said they, " death is not; where death is, we are not. It is the last best boon of nature, for it frees man from all his cares. It is at worst the close of a banquet we have enjoyed". Like the Chinese sages, they confided in the natural goodness of the heart of man, and like the Hindu sages, in the untarnishable nature of his soul. They declared that man was perfectible, and that the perfected man was a divine man and the equal of God. They called themselves sages, and as such claimed to have attained to an impassive tranquillity, or fixed state of philosophical indifference, such as all systems of yoga require and the Eskimos constitutionally possess, and pervaded by which Antoninus Pius, who was one of them, on the last night of his life gave from his deathbed for password of the sentries "equanimity".

Roman Stoicism was the salt that savored the Roman Republic, and under the empire resisted and tempered the tyranny of the rulers and vices of the people until It was overshadowed, or, rather, outshone, by mystical Neoplatonism and early Christian mysticism, and in them sunk and lost to historic view.

CHAPTER XXV - CHRISTIAN YOGA

The Fathers of the Desert

During the first two centuries of Christianity monasticism was unknown; the conditions were much too turbulent, and, besides, the second coming of Jesus was daily-looked for during a good part of that time. But in the third century accident introduced an element of mysticism into the Church that its founders had not thought of, and made sure of its success thenceforth. A refugee from the Decian persecution, known afterwards as Paul the Hermit, fled to the Egyptian desert and hid himself away in one of the tombs dug out of rock which are so numerous there. He was followed by many others, Saint Anthony among them, all of whom became hermits ; soon there was quite a nation of such, and by the close of the next century in a great part of Egypt the monastic population was nearly equal to that of the cities. Away from the churches and priestly control, solitary and in poverty, given to prayer and penance, the refugees found themselves in true yoga conditions, and early began, much to their own surprise and disquiet, no doubt, to have yoga experiences. Dalgairns, a Catholic writer, in his introduction to the authorized account of " The Fathers of the Desert", says of them that the Church " had such onfidence in its own strength and in the loyalty of her children that she allowed them to go out into the wilds and lead a solitary life — allowed them to stray into the desert and plunge into the dangerous depths of contemplation — left them to win their own spiritual experience". Troubled by the stirring within them of those mystical forces common to all men however variously interpreted, the hermits were accustomed to come together and exchange experiences and counsel, until in time some among them became by that means sufficiently instructed to act as teachers of the rest — gurus. The yoga practice thus resulting, in the absence of other mould to receive it, took Christian form, and thus came into being Christian magic, a magic that will be seen to have been a fit adjunct and support to a faith whose chief article is salvation by torture. Mr. Lecky says, in speaking of this movement : " There is, perhaps, no phase in the moral history of mankind of a deeper or more painful interest than this ascetic epidemic. A hideous, sordid and emaciated maniac, without knowledge, without patriotism, without natural affection, passing his life in a long routine of endless self-torture, and quailing before the ghastly phantoms of his delirious brain become the ideal of the nations which had known the writings of Plato and Cicero and the lives of Socrates and Cato. " Again: " Some of the hermits lived in deserted dens of wild beasts, others in dried-up wells, while others found a congenial resting place among the tombs. Some disdained all clothes and crawled abroad like wild beasts, covered only by their matted hair. In Mesopotamia, and part of Syria, there existed a sect known by the name of 'Grazers', who never lived under a roof, who ate neither flesh nor bread, but spent their time forever on the mountain side, and ate grass like cattle. The cleanliness of the body was regarded as a pollution of the soul, and the saints who were most admired had become one hideous mass of clotted filth". The women were no neater than the men, as witness famous Saint Sylvia, who was such a devoted slut that when her own uncleanliness had made her ill, she refused to take the bath prescribed for her cure; witness also Saint Mary of Egypt, once a great beauty, as, naked and blackened with the dirt of forty-seven years' accretion, her tangled hair floating in the wind, she treads along the valley of Moab, and as she passes by a meditating anchorite frightens him into believing her an image of the devil conjured up to mock him. Ignorance seemed to be in as much favor with them as uncleanliness. "The great majority of the early monks appear to have been men who were not only absolutely ignorant themselves, but who also looked on learning with positive disfavor". "The duty of a monk", said Saint Jerome, "is not to teach, but to weep". In weeping, by the way, they were proficient; one of them wept his eyelashes off their lids and wore a cloth on his breast to catch his tears. Many of them kept themselves continually under the pangs of hunger, some taking but one meal every two days, and others but one in a week. For two centuries the craziness lasted, and then the free and wild yoga of the desert, having developed a new element for ecclesiasticism to work upon, and having also become dangerously turbulent, passed under priestly control, and in time became the regulated monasticism that now exists. The same Dalgairns truly asserts that to the fathers of the desert the Church owes its mystical theology, and praises their methods of mortification and prayer, as being still obligatory on good Catholics. His words are these: "There is no possible Christian life but in the old path of mortification and prayer". He makes, too, the singular admission that the yoga methods of the desert were essentially the same as those of the Neoplatonists; he says: " Neoplatonism was a doctrine of which the end and object was union with God; and though their god was impersonal, yet their system was a real mysticism of which the climax was ecstasy. Proclus also, in his books on the Theology of Plato, and Plotinus himself, in many places, speak much of ecstasy and of abstraction from the things of sense, in a way not contrary to the maxims of Christian wisdom". Again, the author of "The Heavenly Wisdom according to the Egyptians" thus writes of himself: "I often, when engaged in mental contemplation, seem to leave my body and to enjoy the possession of the highest good with marvellous delight". "Wherein", says Dalgairns, "did this system of union with God differ from that of St. Anthony ? "

But it did differ, and widely. As regards methods, the Neoplatonist was not bound to any religious observance, affiliation or declaration of faith, nor need he renounce the world, live in poverty or as a celibate, torment his flesh or go dirty, while as to the state of absorption he aimed at, it was, if less complete than that of a Hindu Yoga, far more so than that the Christian ascetic could hope for, and with a God as different from Jehovah as a principle is from a person. Dalgairns gives as a reason why the methods of the desert were better than those of the Neoplatonists that the latter had to be both learned men and philosophers. But if the fact that without being either, the anchorites attained to ecstasy and union with their god proves that neither learning nor philosophy could have been essential, the other fact that the philosophers got to theirs without being Christians, hermits, ascetics celibates or paupers, without self-torment, vermin or dirt, proves that no more were any of these essential. Clearly, then, neither was the only way. The Christian Church has long since discovered that dirt and vermin are not nice nor necessary means of grace, though penance remains still in vogue. All three of them are offences against the human body; and the human body it is that yoga practice most manifestly works upon, the earliest results being its improved health and beauty, and into it flow and along its nerves play the vibrations so often mentioned in the Church writings as "bliss, sweetness, the sweetness of the flesh", etc. An ascetic absorbed in devotion may easily fall into slovenly ways, but the saints of the desert were slovenly on religious principle. The Essenes wore their garments to rags, but kept clean skins. So do Hindu Yogis now, unless perchance they be of the sect of Jains, who, believing all life to be divine and therefore sacred, will not wash or scratch themselves lest they should kill vermin or animalculae. These, too, are dirty on a religious principle, but a different one from that of the Christians, who believed divine favor could be got by bodily discomfort and cutaneous disease per se. These were to them modes of penance, and penance being a sacrament of their church, sacramental too were fleas and the itch. But uncleanness cannot possess any magical value, since it cannot be supposed to aid concentration. It is otherwise with pain, and such bloody self-flagellations as Saint John of the Cross and Saint Theresa were addicted to, had doubtless a certain value in helping them on their way, for pain compels concentration even to the extent of inducing the trance state which in turn kills it, as in the cases of martyrs hereinbefore alluded to. Admitting this, we may also admit that for such devotees as are too indolent or stupid to acquire the requisite con centration in any pleasanter way painful inflictions may have their use, and though futile as a means of pleasing God, may be effective in fixing the mind. But this could be the case only in the earlier of the two stages into which, as will be seen, Christian mystics divide the saint's progress, namely meditation; in the later one, that of contemplation, it could hardly prove other than a distraction.

St. John of the Cross

How Christian mysticism, thus strangely originating in the wilderness, afterwards in the keeping of the church took shape and development is well shown in the lately republished life and writings of Saint John of the Cross, already mentioned, a work of high authority. He was indeed an able man, who in the midst of his maniacal austerities could dissect and analyze his own abnormal sensations, visions and ideas with a strong hand and clear head, and note down and classify them in a way that makes his book of great service to the modern student of things occult. By his time monasticism had lost much of the severity of its earlier centuries, and probably all of the untidiness the fathers of the desert carried into it. Nothing in the account of his life which the book contains tells of his being unclean, however much matured. On the contrary, it affirms with detail that the rags from his sores were regularly washed, and by ladies of rank who disputed with one another for privilege to do so, in a rivalry made the more eager by the fact that the linen had a true odor of sanctity. But the mitigation of the original austerities of the order of Carmelites to which he belonged, which mitigation had obtained general acceptance, did not at all please one who could wear about his waist a barbed iron chain plus a sackcloth shirt and do with but two hours of sleep in a night, and John of the Cross went all lengths with his coadjutor the nun Theresa, in making the practice conform to the old rule, in getting back to the usages of the times when the brethren of Saint Mary first left the world "to live in caves and hollows of the rocks intent on the service of God and their own salvation". Of the nun it is told that she would flog her white back till the red blood sprinkled the walls of her cell, and of the monk that "through the silence of the night the sound of his lash would reach the ears of the friars, who trembled when they heard it, for they knew how merciless he was to himself". What is strange is that both of them seemed to like it, seemed to have in some way got so hungry for it that it must have lost all virtue as a penance and become a sinful indulgence. In fact John of the Cross, in denouncing certain innovations in the direction of increased severity, seems himself to have thought as much. He gave as a reason against them that the young friars "would be carried away by the sweetness of excessive penance and miss the road to solid devotion". Again he says of such " gluttons " as he terms them, "Allured by the sweetness they find therein, some of them kill themselves with penance". Being at one time a prisoner in the keeping of his opposers, the Friars of the Mitigation, he was each evening at supper time brought into the refectory, and scourged on his bare shoulders in a way that marked him for life. But he took the scourging with such evident satisfaction that his tormentors got tired of it and desisted. " This was to him another grief; he complained to his gaoler, and asked him why he was forgotten and deprived of his only consolation". All which is hard to understand unless we can suppose that practice thoroughly and long persisted in, has power, along with other bodily modifications it effects, such as adamantine hardness, control of breath, levitation, Herculean strength, etc., to actually reverse the normal action of the sensory nerves and convert pain into pleasure, or else so completely overcome pain by pleasure that none is felt, which last, by the way, would hardly be more strange than that a condemned witch could tranquilly slumber on a pile of burning fagots, a thing that has often happened.

The miraculous experiences of John of the Cross begun early in his boyhood. He fell into a deep pool, but floated on the surface, and was rescued without needing to accept the extended hand of a suddenly appearing beautiful visionary lady. He fell into a well, but was received in the arms of a like apparition, so that he took no hurt. The voice of the Lord was heard by him, both inwardly and by his outer ear. Called to confess a nun, and finding her dead, he prayed her back to life, and kept her so long enough to be shrived: and then she died a second time. He and Theresa, while conversing in the convent parlor, were both raised in the air, the monk on one side of the bars and the nun on the other; and at all times he was liable to be entranced and lifted up on the slightest provocation, such as the singing of a verse of a hymn. A nun tempted by a spirit of blasphemy, uncleanness and doubt was relieved by his ministrations ; but as soon as he left her, the Devil assumed his form and went and re-confessed her on his own account. When the friar discovered this he made sure it should not again occur by writing out and signing his instructions. But soon came a letter, as from him, that again reversed them, and which was so well forged that when shown it he declared it was his own handwriting and signature. The Devil then was taken in hand and regularly exorcised. But he played the same prank with another penitent, from whom he had obtained a written contract that she would be his bride as his recompense for having conferred on her the gift of tongues. Again exorcised, he confessed and gave up the contract. Here was no victory for John of the Cross, for the Devil prevailed until the power of the Church was called in, but Saint Theresa wrote that he had put to flight three legions of devils, whom, in the name of God, he commanded to tell their number, and was obeyed on the instant. Just before he escaped from prison his cell was brightly and supernaturally illuminated, and the Lord's voice was heard promising he should be set free, which was soon done, the Virgin Mary herself showing him the way out. Again, while praying before a picture of Jesus a voice came from it saying: " John, what shall I give thee for all thou hast done and suffered for me?" He was able to read the secret thoughts of his penitents, reminding them of sins they had forgotten or fraudulently omitted to confess. Finally, he calmed a tempest, extinguished a conflagration, and obtained a supply of food, all by his prayers. With all these gifts he died in disgrace, stripped of all his offices, but that was what he liked, and had prayed for. Humility is an important condition to yoga practice, for the reason that it is the opposite to self-conceit, which is a sad hindrance to concentration, as is well recognized by both Chinese and Hindu authorities. John of the Cross, to be sure, knew nothing of Chinese or Hindu Yoga, but as a Christian he held to the promise of Jesus, that " he who humbleth himself shall be exalted", and humbled himself accordingly. The reward he received must have exceeded his highest expectations, for his departure was honored with prodigies such as any saint might be proud of. Just before he died there appeared a great orb of light encircling him, " which was so brilliant as to dim the other lights in the room and the candles on the altar", and on the Monday night following the funeral, his brethren being assembled as usual for discipline in the darkened church, "were suddenly surprised by a great light which filled the whole church. Some thought that all the lights had not been put out, and the prior gave orders in that sense, but those who were near the grave were seized with a holy fear, for they saw that it had come from the tomb of the saint, whose sepulchre it had pleased our Lord to make thus glorious before their eyes. In a few minutes the light disappeared". Nine months after interment, upon his grave being opened, the body was found incorrupt, perfectly fresh and supple, giving out a most fragrant perfume. When one devotee, to obtain a relic, cut off a finger, the hand bled freely, and when another attempted to do the same it was jerked out of his grasp. A piece of the flesh kept in a glass jar took on a good likeness of the saint, and conjured up to the eyes of many persons, at many different times visions of the Virgin and Child, of Christ on the cross, of John himself, Peter and other saints, besides Elijah the Prophet and many angels. And so died John of the Cross, after making as many people as he could as uncomfortable as he could, died glorying in his humility and in an odor of sanctity peculiar, penetrating and persistent.

The Writings of St. John of the Cross

The voluminous work that he left behind him was written, as he tells us, at the request and for the benefit of "only certain persons of our holy order of Mount Carmel of the primitive observance". It was, therefore, like the Upanishads of the Hindus, written by a yogi and for the instruction of yogis. It is nothing less than a manual of Christian yoga, by which devotees may be led along the path to what he terms "the high state of perfection, called here union of the soul with God" ; again, "the perfect union of the love of God" ; again, "being transformed in God; because he communicates his own supernatural being in such a way that the soul seems to be God himself and to possess the things of God. The soul seems to be God rather than itself, and indeed is God by participation, though in reality preserving its own natural substance as distinct from God as it did before". But to show how little the approachment here indicated is from the identification, absorption or assimilation of other systems, we have: "But remember that among all creatures, the highest and the lowest, there is not one that comes near unto God. For, though it be true, as theologians tell us, that all creatures bear a certain relation to God, and are tokens of his being, some more, some less, according to the greater or less perfection of their nature, yet there is no essential likeness or communion between them and him; yea, rather the distance between His divine nature and their nature is infinite". No stronger words than these are needed to distinguish the end and aim of Christian yoga from the end and aim of every other. Connected with the state, whatever it may be, that is here termed union with God, much is said about ecstatic "touches" of knowledge and sweetness given by Him, that are so strong and profound as "to penetrate into the innermost substance of the soul". For there are some acts of knowledge and touches of God wrought by Him in the substance of the soul which so enrich it that one of them is sufficient, not only to purge away at once certain imperfections which had hitherto resisted the efforts of a whole life, but also to fill the soul with virtues and divine gifts. Such is the sweetness and deep delight of these touches of God, that one of them is more than a recompense for all the sufferings of this life, however great their number. "Sometimes the touches are surprises, coming when the soul is occupied with something else, at times coming gently and at times so as to make "not only the soul, but the body also, to tremble". They are, it is furthermore stated, "a part of the union " — are "touches of union".

The external conditions proper to the practice of Christian Yoga are poverty, seclusion and solitude, and the internal ones detachment, devotion and humility, while the practical methods are religious observance, prayer, fasting, penance, meditation and spiritual contemplation. All of these are found in Hindu Yoga. Poverty, seclusion and solitude are easily seen to be important aids, if not essential ones, to concentration; so is devotion, itself a mode of concentration; so is humility, as neutralizing self-conceit and giving receptivity, while detachment, which means the not setting the heart on things of this life, whether possessing them or not, is a mental state of evident importance. Complete detachment is an absolute cut-off from temptations and disturbances of every sort. Prayer, fasting and other religious observance serve as helps to, or even as substitutes for, concentration; but while the Hindu who has by means of them "attained" is thereby released from them all, the Christian ascetic never is done with any of them, his religion never letting go her grip on his magic; and since the time of St. Benedict the Church no longer allows " the yells of the wild Egyptian monks to disturb the propriety of her councils", but holds her ascetics securely controlled in monasteries and nunneries. Other methods of yoga practice include among their austerities self-inflicted penance of the kind calling for passive endurance and intended to induce and also test the virtue of equanimity, the flower of stoical philosophy; but in Christian Yoga penance plays a much larger part, because, as said before, Christian religion adds another motive to it, namely, the desire to please God by displeasing ourselves. In early Christian times, when Adam's fall, hell's fire and redemption by crucifixion were about the sum and substance of the new religion, there must have been ever present in believers' minds the idea of torment, tending to breed there a morbid taste for it and a disposition to supplement Christ's sufferings with their own, so that the measure of his Father's wrath might not merely be kept full but made to run over, and a desire in each of them to have a cross and passion of his own. Thus when the refugees from persecution took to the desert, their religious exercise consisted of prayer and penance only. " They anticipated no contemplation", says Dalgairns. So that as their prayers were brief and few their devotions must have been chiefly made up of hurting themselves in diverse ways, until the favoring conditions of enforced solitude and idleness let in meditation and contemplation and made involuntary yogis of them. John of the Cross distinguishes meditation from the succeeding stage of contemplation as follows: "The difference between these two conditions of the soul is like the difference between working and enjoyment of the fruit of our work; between receiving a gift and profiting by it; between the toil of travelling and the rest at our journey's end ; between the preparation of our food and the eating or enjoyment of it. If the soul be not occupied either with its bodily faculties in meditation and reflection, or with its spiritual faculties in contemplation or pure knowledge, it is impossible to say that it is occupied at all". He then tells the signs by which it may be known that the time has come to pass from meditation to contemplation; they are present when it becomes irksome to meditate, or when there is disinclination to fix the imagination or the senses on particular objects, but more distinctly when the soul delights to be alone, waiting lovingly on God, without any particular considerations, in interior peace, quiet and repose, where the acts and exercises of the understanding, memory and will, at least discursively — which is the going from one subject to another — have ceased; nothing remains except that knowledge and attention, general and loving, of which I have spoken, without the particular perception of aught else". Till these signs appear it is better to continue practicing meditation, and even after quitting it, it is sometimes well to return to it. Of the nature of contemplation, it is trance. A state of trance in which the soul receives divine knowledge is thus described: "The soul seems unconscious of all it knows, and is therefore lost, as it were, in forgetfulness, knowing not where it is, nor what has happened to it, unaware of the lapse of time. It may and does occur that many hours pass while it is in this state of forgetfulness; all seems to last but a moment when it again returns to itself. The cause of this forgetfulness is the pureness and simplicity of this knowledge, which, being itself pure and clear, cleanses the soul while it fills it, and purifies it of all the apprehensions and forms of sense and memory through which it once acted and thus brings it to a state of forgetfulness and unconsciousness of the flight of time. The prayer of the soul, though in reality long, lasts but for a moment, because it is an act of pure intelligence". John of the Cross was often in such trances, and wrote from his own experiences.

Concerning the revelations which come by way of such deep contemplation, he says: " Some supernatural knowledge is corporeal, and some spiritual. The former is of two kinds: one of them enters the understanding through the exterior bodily senses ; and the other through the interior bodily senses, comprehending all that the imagination may grasp, form and conceive. The spiritual supernatural knowledge is also of two kinds: one distinct and special; the other confused, obscure and general. The first kind comprises four particular apprehensions, communicated to the mind without the intervention of any one of the bodily senses. These are visions, revelations, locutions and spiritual impressions. The second kind, which is obscure and general, has but one form, that of contemplation, which is the work of faith. The soul is to be led into this by directing it thereto through all the rest, beginning with the first, and detaching it from them " (one by one). Of the supernatural "apprehensions " just named, the following are instances: "They (spiritual men) sometimes see the forms and figures of those of another life, saints, or angels, good and evil, or certain extraordinary lights and brightness.

They hear strange words, sometimes seeing those who utter them, and sometimes not. They have a sensible perception at times of most sweet odors, without knowing whence they proceed. Their sense of taste is also deliciously affected; and that of the touch so sweetly caressed at times that the bones and the marrow exult and rejoice, bathed as it were in joy". But all these, for many reasons, which he elaborates, one of which is that the devil can produce them as well as God, we must reject and disregard. "The soul must close its eyes on and reject them, come they whence they may — unless in certain rare instances, after examination by a learned spiritual and experienced director. " But John of the Cross speaks only for himself. A church that cackles with triumph as often as a miraculous tgg is laid within her fold is not the institution to sanction the flinging overboard of a cargo of evidences of Christianity having virtue sufficient to establish an hundred religions and an hundred heresies, as such things go.

Next in order in the devotee's spiritual experience are locutions, or words supernaturally produced, without the instrumentality of the bodily senses, and designated as successive, formal and substantial. Successive words come to the mind when it is absorbed in a given subject, and then it " puts words and reasonings together so much to the purpose, and with such facility and clearness discovers by reflection things it knew not before, that it seems to itself as if it were not itself which did so, but some third person which addressed it interiorly, reasoning, answering and informing ; the mind then reasons with itself as one man with another". "He who is in this state cannot believe that the words do not proceed from some third person". The disposition prevailing in his day even among those who had hardly begun to meditate, to accept such words as coming from God filled our saint with terror. "But", says he, "it is not true; such an one has only been speaking to himself". The words may come from the Holy Spirit, the devil, or the natural light of the understanding, and it is hard to tell which, but there should be no account made of any of them " from whatever source they may come". Formal words are such as the mind" formally perceives to be spoken by a third person independently of its own operations, without any effort on its part, sometimes even when the mind is not recollected, and is far from thinking what is uttered within it, which is not the case with successive words, which always relate to a matter which then occupies the mind". These, too, may come either from God or the devil. Before acting upon them the confessor must be consulted and "no soul who does not deal with them as with an enemy" is safe from delusions. Substantial words execute themselves — are acts of God and not merely commands or instructions. Thus when he spoke these to Abraham, "Walk before me and be perfect", Abraham was by the very fact of their utterance made perfect; it was not his to accept or reject them. The saint informs us that neither the understanding of man nor the arts of the devil can simulate substantial words.

Next in order come "spiritual impressions", which are of two degrees of excellence, both acting directly on the will. "Neither the soul that receives them, nor its director can ever know their sources, or why God effects them ; they do not depend in any way on good works or meditation". They are caused by "touches of union " with God, are " most intense, high, profound, and secret, and seem not to touch the will, but to have been wrought in the very substance of the soul", and from them "there flows frequently into the understanding the apprehension of knowledge or intelligence which is usually a most profound and secret sense of God, to which, as well as to the impression from which it flows, no name can be given". Yet even here, he says, there is danger of delusion and need of caution ; "the understanding ought not to meddle with them, but remain passive, inclining the will to consent freely and gratefully, and not interfering itself".

Stupidity

The saint has much to say in relation to "the purgation and active night of the memory and the will", and of the annihilation of both powers, in the matter of their operation, in respect to all knowledge whether of natural or supernatural objects. Beginning with natural knowledge, he says: " The memory must be stripped and emptied of it all; it must labor to destroy all sense of it, so that no impression whatever shall be left behind". And again : "The more the memory is united to God the more it loses all distinct knowledge, and at last all such fades utterly away when the state of perfection is reached. In the beginning, when this is going on, great forgetfulness ensues; men neglect themselves in outward things, forgetting to eat and drink. But he who has attained to the habit of union is able to attend to the duties of life by means of knowledge supplied in a special way by God, the operation of the memory and of the other powers being in that state, as it were, divine. God has entered into possession". To illustrate the methods by which one so possessed is directed the following is offered: "A perfect man has at a certain time a certain indispensable business to transact. He has no recollection whatever of it, but in some way he knows not, it will present itself to his mind, through that stirring of his memory of which I speak, at the time and in the way it ought, and that without fail". Supernatural knowledge is equally with natural a danger and a hindrance, and " visions and revelations, locutions and impressions" must all be rigorously emptied out and carefully kept out of memory. " It is therefore necessary for the soul to forget and detach itself from all distinct forms and knowledge of supernatural things, that it may not hinder in the memory the divine union in perfect hope. " Having shown how to purify the memory, the saint next considers the will, which, he says, must be purged of all its affections or passions, namely, of joy, hope, grief and fear, "Man must feel no joy except for that which is simply for the honor and glory of our Lord God, nor hope except in him, nor grief except in what concerns him, nor fear but of him only", and he quotes from one Boethius: "Wilt thou contemplate truth in a clear light? Drive away joy and hope and grief and fear". All which shows that no system of yoga practice can go further than the Christian in the thoroughness of its detachment and renunciation.

The Horrors

The next step on the way to sainthood brings the practicer to the stage which our teacher names "the dark night". This night — it is contemplation — produces two sorts of darkness or purgation, the first of which, the night of sense, in which the soul is purified or detached from things of sense, is the lot of many; the second, in which it is purified and detached in the spirit and prepared for union with God, is the lot of very few and is little spoken or written about, or even known by experience. In this night are the well-known religious "horrors" common to Protestants and Catholics alike. The night of sense is bitter and terrible to the senses, but the night of spirit is incomparably more awful to the spirit. Souls begin to enter the dark night when God is drawing them out of the state of beginners, or those who meditate, and is leading them into that of proficients, or those who contemplate, in order that, having passed through this, they may arrive at the state of union with God, which is that of the perfect. In the dark night the practicer finds himself unable to advance a single step in meditation as before, the inward sense being overwhelmed and abandoned to dryness so great that he has no longer joy or sweetness in his spiritual exercises, finding nothing in their place but insipidity and bitterness. All his own efforts are now in vain, for he is being led by another and different road, that of contemplation. But, with all this, there will in due course come a consciousness of strength and energy; and this is the commencement of contemplation, which in this stage is generally secret and goes on unknown to him who is being acted on, and by the dryness and emptiness it produces in the senses makes him long for solitude and quiet, without the power of reflecting on anything distinctly, or even desiring to do so. In this state he should know how to be quiet, to disregard every exterior or interior work, to be without solicitude for anything, and resign himself into the hands of God, keeping his soul tranquil, for were he now to exert his interior faculties they would only hinder and ruin the good which God is working to his soul. Among the spiritual "imperfections" of beginners are pride, avarice, anger, envy, gluttony and luxury. In treating of this last the saint discloses experiences of a peculiar nature, and which must be noted here, that later they may be considered and compared with like experiences in other yogas. He says that practicers very often, in the midst of their spiritual exercises, and when they cannot help themselves, feel the impure movements of sensuality, and sometimes even when their minds are absorbed in prayer, or when they are receiving the sacrament of penance and the eucharist.

And, to the great disgust of the soul, even when it has made some progress, with the spiritual delight that flows into it the sensual part occasionally mingles its own delight. Sometimes it is Satan who sets up the rebellious movements in order to disgust the soul during prayer, causing some to relax in prayer, and some to abandon it altogether, being more liable to these assaults during prayer than at other times. This is not all, for he represents before them then most vividly the most foul and filthy images. " Some are so grievously assailed that they dare not dwell upon anything, lest it become at once a stumbling-block to them". A third source of these depraved movements is the very fear of them. But, when the sensual part is renewed in the purgation of the dark night, such afflictions disappear, and as the love of God grows in the soul the human love cools and is forgotten.

The Night of the Spirit

Having undergone the purgations of the night of sense the soul attains to the state of proficients where it finds itself able to rise at will to the most tranquil and loving contemplation, and have joy and spiritual sweetness without the fatigue of meditation. But it does not at once enter into union with God; it must spend some time, perhaps years, in the exercises of that state. And then there is yet a further purgation to undergo, that of the night of the spirit, without which the intercourse of the proficient with God is still most mean. In that night the faculties, affections and feelings, spiritual and sensual, interior and exterior, must be denuded, leaving the understanding in darkness, the will dry, the memory empty, the affections of the soul in the deepest affliction, bitterness and distress; all which is effected in the soul by means of contemplation pure and dark. And this contemplation is not a night, a darkness merely, but pain and torment as well. It is called infused contemplation, or mystical theology, and in it the practicer is, according to the saint, taught by God the truths of the Catholic religion, without effort on his part, and in a secret, hidden way in which the natural operations of the understanding have no share. Many reasons are given why the process is called dark and why it is painful, but the reasons, as well as the facts they relate to, are purely religious, and applicable only to Christian ascetics. The valley of horrors trod by the Christian pilgrim on his way to his God would, of course, be different from that trod by a Hindu one on his way to his. But, besides religious horrors, practicers of all faiths must needs go through many "sloughs of despond" in their long and hard journey; and, moreover, yoga being an affair of the body, physical pangs must be expected as well by all. The first effect of yoga practice is to put the body in good condition, which, if disease be present, often involves an aggravation of its symptoms, they being merely nature's curative efforts. In this last stage of the saint's progress all effects are operated through love, and knowledge and belief only come in by way of the heart. In his "Spiritual Canticle of the Soul and the Bridegroom Christ" and "Living Flame of Love", and his voluminous commentaries on them which cover 350 octavo pages, John of the Cross, inadvertently perhaps, emulates Solomon in saying one thing and meaning another, in treating of divine love in terms of human love. Of his writings it may be said that they not only identify Christian sanctity with Hindu and other yoga, but embody a large number of experiences of great scientific value.

Postel

Contemporary with John of the Cross was Guillaume Postel, a French monk and physician, one of the most learned men of the time. Crowds of students attended his teaching at the College of Lombards in Paris, and it was said of him that there came out of his mouth as many oracles as words. But though in high favor with the great, he was accused by theologians of deism and atheism because he claimed to be able to prove the Christian religion to be true by reason alone and asserted that by means of reason, without aid of faith, he would himself convert the whole world. He claimed, moreover, that all the truths of nature were written in Hebrew characters on the sky formed by the arrangement of the stars, and that he had read them there ; and also that the Kabala had revealed to him that the world would last but six thousand years longer, and that before the end man would recover his primitive state of innocence and happiness. His conduct was correct, his life pure above reproach, and his benevolence wide. During several years he was confessor to a Venetian nun named Mother Jeanne, of great repute for sanctity, and abounding in spiritual gifts, of the order John of the Cross held to be untrustworthy, such as visions, revelations, transfiguration, etc. Already possessed by the idea of woman's supremacy, he easily fell under her control, and in his newly devised religious system made her the chief character as the incarnation of the spirit of Jesus Christ and the mother regenerator of all mankind; reserving to himself the spiritual headship of the new church to be made up of the Jews and all Christian sects, including the Mohammedans, united in one fold, and which all others were to be invited to enter on pain of death, and according to the King of France the temporal empire of all the nations of the earth united in peace.

Pursuant to a promise the nun made to him she came to him after she died ; as he expressed it : " She kept her word. She came to me in Paris, she illumined me with her light, she reconciled my reason with my faith. Her substance and spiritual body two years after her ascension to heaven descended into me, and extended themselves throughout my sensible body, so that it is she and not I that lives in me". Concerning her appearance as he knew her in life he says that, though more than fifty years old, she would pass for fifteen, especially when taking the communion; and of his own, after she took possession of him as above, it is related that his pale, old wrinkled visage became smooth and rosy and his white locks became black.

To obtain spirituality Postel prescribed, besides very fervent prayer, very devout meditation and very vehement contemplation, and in distinguishing the one from the other, says: "Meditation is when one holds his thought a long time on a word, a proposition, or a fact, or a beneficence of our Lord, in considering his infinite mercy, power, wisdom, pity, justice, virtue, glory and other perfect qualities, or, on the other hand, on man's infinite wickedness, felony, weakness, ignorance, avarice, vice, injustice", etc. — or, best of all, the suffering of Jesus, dwelling on which, one hour, or even one minute, is worth more than a thousand years' time bestowed on any other subject.

"And what", he asks, "is contemplation?" "It is known to but few and is very difiicult to make understood, but by similitudes it may be explained. Just as the doctrine of metaphysics treats of natural things without considering the words, bodies or images of them which are in the mind, but by considering them by their essences, abstract and wholly separate from body, so also should contemplation do. Meditation must pass into contemplation when the soul would force itself to know and feel God in all nature, so that only the sovereign cause of all things is perceived there, which is essence, unity, truth and divine goodness", and "seeing in all things the spirit of God". In fine, contemplation is nothing else than reducing all objects into divine beauty, and the passion of God into the infinite love whence it proceeds, as much that love which is intellectual and high as into that which is low, animal and sensual. Postel closed his life in enforced seclusion, and after signing as many recantations as were laid before him.

Quietism

In the following century rose the sect known as Quietists, of which Miguel Molinos, another Spanish priest, was the head and Madame Guyon the most famous disciple. Possibly Quietism was the most seductive heresy that ever troubled Rome, whither Molinos early in his career went for the purpose of preaching it, and whence it rapidly spread throughout all Catholic countries, gaining adherents among the highest church dignitaries, including the Pope himself. In Naples alone there were 20,000 who followed the "new method", as it was called. In it religious observances had so small a part, and its good fruits were so evident, that the Jesuits became alarmed and resolved to suppress it. They tried polemics at first. A book written by one of them took the ground that though Quietism in itself was good, its practice led to evil. The Quietist was too good for this rude, brawling world, and this new method, however useful to very pious souls, was not fitted for the every-day life of the ordinary Christian. But so strong had Quietism already become that the writer of the polemic was condemned by the Inquisition and his book put in the Index. The Jesuits, however, became all the more eager to put down the rising heresy, and brought influences to bear which finally caused the Inquisition to arrest Molinos, try and condemn him, despite his powerfnl supporters. He escaped being burnt by making public abjuration, and so was allowed to live out his life in prison. Equally energetic action elsewhere suppressed the movement completely. Viewed as merely a religious modification, Quietism is briefly but well described by Bishop Burnet, thus: " The substance of the whole is reduced to this, that, in our prayers and other devotions, the best methods are to retire the mind from all gross images, and so to form an act of faith, and thereby to present ourselves before God, and then to sink into silence and cessation of new acts, and to let God act upon us, and so to follow His conduct. This way Molinos preferred to the multiplication of new acts and other forms of devotion, and he makes small account of corporeal austerities and reduces all the exercises of religion to this simplicity of mind. He thinks this is not only to be proposed to religious houses, but even to secular persons". Just here was the offence of Molinos, He undertook to popularize the methods of sanctification discovered by the fathers of the desert and well known to the Church, but in practice confined to cloistered persons only, and to that end had mitigated and simplified them so that all could practice them. Confined to monasteries and nunneries, the eccentricities and enthusiasms" of the yogis and yoginis could be controlled or hidden, and even made to do service to the Church, which had, however, too good a recollection of the disturbances made in earlier times by those same fathers to let yoga again get loose in the Catholic world. Secular persons might well enough be fed by their spiritual directors with such moderate portions of that magical ecstasy which goes by the name of religious comfort and consolation as a daily round of religious observances, fastings, repetitions and other lulling monotonies, and occasional "retreats" might procure them, and yet be kept in order. But to allow them to help themselves, to allow God to act as confessor and spiritual director, to open a postern door free to all in Saint Peter's own gate, would be quite another thing. The Quietists lived exemplary lives and were happy in their religion, but they were indifferent as to religious observance. They seldom went to mass or confession, or made pilgrimages, did but scanty penance, cared little for images or relics, and spent little money for praying out of purgatory their dead relations. Such a movement as theirs must needs be dangerous to any church, because dangerous to religion itself. Had it been allowed to go on the religious appendages to contemplation would one after another have been found to be non-essential and dropped, until finally there would have remained only Quietism pure and simple, that is to say yoga pure and simple. Assuredly, then, the Jesuits were wise in their generation. How far their wisdom would avail them in this generation is another question. The Holy Inquisition is no more!

Although greatly mitigated in severity, the instructions of Molinos to his penitents were essentially the same as those of John of the Cross to his. The practicer must be "quiet from fears, void of affections, desires and thoughts, must work, pray, obey and suffer without being the least moved". For penance the ordinary miseries of human life would serve, but he must expect to go through seasons of darkness and dryness, and, when "God intends to guide him in an extraordinary manner", as in the case of Madame Guyon, be prepared to endure extraordinary suffering. In her detail of experiences she says: "The soul thus in corruption is so full of horror at itself that it cannot endure itself. The pain of suffering its own stench is so great that it is no longer concerned at anything that can be done to it outwardly. Nothing any longer affects it. It sees itself worthy of all scorn. Others see it only with horror", " It plunges into putrefaction as into the place appropriate to it", " Well, perhaps this corruption will last but a little while. Alas! quite otherwise. It will last several years". " At length, by slow degrees, the soul gets used to its corruption, and it becomes natural to it, except at certain times, when it exhales a stench enough to cause its death, were it not immortal". And even to the ordinary penitent Molinos says: "Know, however, that thou art to be plunged in a bitter sea of sorrow, and of internal and external pains, which torments will pierce into the most inward part of thy soul and body". Certainly in all hereinbefore summarized of pagan yoga there has been no mention made of any such horrors as these. The worst that can happen to a Hindu practicer, for example, if he fail to make connection with his Brahman, is to go on with his re-incarnations, and in some future one try again ; but the Christian, hanging by the slender thread of faith between heaven's dome and hell's pit, a cruel devil below and an angry God above, when he does get discouraged must needs get horridly so.

In connection with his mitigation of the severity of the old cloistered yoga devised to adapt it to the world at large, Molinos relied on a peculiar method of so starting the penitent on his way that the growth of his soul in sanctity should go of itself, despite disturbing cares and avocations, "if he will walk in continual and virtual praying and strive to acquire a habit of internal recollection, defined to mean ' faith and silence in the presence of God". The mode of starting was as follows: "Thou oughtest to go to prayer that thou mayest deliver thyself wholly up into the hands of God, with perfect resignation, exerting an act of faith, believing thou art in the divine presence, afterwards settling in that holy repose with quietness, silence, tranquillity; and endeavoring for a whole day, a whole year, and thy whole life to continue that first act of contemplation by faith and love ". Then if his thoughts should wander, he is encouraged by these words: " So long as thou retractest not that faith and intention of being resigned to God, thou walkest in faith and resignation and consequently in prayer and in virtual and acquired contemplation, although thou perceive it not". Virtual prayer and contemplation seem but feeble means for raising the soul up to union with God, however they may have appeared to produce the expected results, because followed by them. But the reader .who bears in mind what has been said concerning Hindu and Chinese Yoga will be apt to find the cause of such results in that measure of actual contemplation which is compatible with a busy life, and is even found in doing the duties of such a life, as in the cases of the Chinese cook and armorer and the Indian butcher and overworked woman of all work, who did their work with concentrated minds, and thereby became more or less of yogis.

Molinos describes the progress of the penitent as being along a path wherein, step by step, he is led by God, to whose guidance he must absolutely yield himself, happen what may. Concerning the passing from meditation into contemplation, he says: "The soul then that is entered into internal recollection hath no need to enter by the first door of meditation on the mysteries, being always taken up in meditating on them, because that is not to be done without great fatigue to the intellect, nor does it stand in need of such ratiocinations, since these serve only as a means to attaining to believing that which it hath already got possession of".

Martin Luther

Every great religious movement may be presumed to have been made by a mystic, that is to say, by a yogi of some degree of attainment, until the contrary is shown. Such an one was Martin Luther. It was as a Catholic monk, shut within his cell, agonized with persistent religious horrors, inventing continually new forms of penance, tormenting himself to death, as he expressed it, to make his peace with God, that he developed the ability to hear a voice that told him to found his church on justification by faith, and to have clear visions of the devil. But this ceased when he became an avowed Protestant and had to go out into the world and strive with his opposers, so that he hardly got further on the path than Mohammed did. And he discarded monasticism, fasts, vigils and penances and other practices promotive of mental concentration, while as to the visions, voices and other mystical phenomena which concentration is apt to produce, the spiritual impressions, trances, etc., he disposed of them all by roundly announcing to the world that the age of miracles was past. Thus he severed religion from magic, its mother, and made Protestantism an orphan from its birth. Had he instead of this supplanted monasticism by Quietism, Protestantism might have become something more than a mode of disintegration and decay.

Paracelsus

There are some who discover in the alchemists only secret practicers of yoga, who under terms of chemistry hid their teachings from all but their own kind, and not only never made a grain of gold, but never attempted it, nor were chemists at all. Others strenuously contend that they did actually produce real gold in quantities so large that one of them furnished a king of

England with the means of carrying on a foreign war and another instituted and maintained in the city of Paris many charitable houses.

Should it ever be demonstrated that the occult powers invoked by our Spiritualists have performed the wonder called materialization even to the extent of producing a spray of geranium, the contention may resolve itself into a compromise which, admitting the gold, but denying the chemistry, shall attribute the result to materialization. And then the alchemists will appear as well advanced yogis, who, not caring to be detected in working unauthorized miracles in times when burning at the stake was yet in vogue, pretended to be smelting and distilling in the seclusion of their laboratories, while in fact they were only meditating and contemplating for the purpose of acquiring magical powers. In any case their writings, which disclose nothing save an intent to disclose nothing, are of small value in the present research. But there has lived one alchemist who was not of these. Paracelsus was born in 1483, and was therefore a contemporary of Luther, to whom and to whose reform he was friendly, though not taking any part in the latter, for he was above all sects, because above all religions, unless magic, which was to him all in all, be religion. None of the sects, he said, possessed intellectually the true religion, which was yet to appear in the world. This gives great value to his teachings, delivered as they were from a free and independent mind, for which public opinion had no terrors. Though well educated, he had little esteem for books, and sought knowledge of men and things by associating with all manner of men and handling all sorts of things, and going about on foot in out-ofthe-way places, doing good wherever he went, for he was a good man withal — no man could be hungry for knowledge as he was without a sympathetic and unselfish nature. Thus constituted, he stands forth as the first great magician of Europe who held his knowledge in trust, as it were, for the good of all, and kept nothing secret that it was safe to promulgate.

Paracelsus was an avowed magician. As such he claimed to have discovered important secrets of nature and obtained healing power. He says: "Magic is a teacher of medicine far preferable to all written books. Magic alone (that can neither be conferred by the universities nor created by the awarding of diplomas, but which comes from God) is the true teacher, preceptor and pedagogue, to teach the art of curing the sick. As the physical forms and colors of objects, or as the letters of a book can be seen by the physical eye, likewise the essence and character of all things may be recognized and become known by the inner sense of the soul. I have reflected a great deal upon the magical powers of the soul of man, and I have discovered a great many secrets in nature, and I will tell you that he only could be a true physician who has acquired this power", The means of doing which he says are prayer, or strong desire or aspiration, and exalted imagination and absolute faith in the omnipotence of the power within ourselves. "The great world is only the product of the universal mind, and man is a little world of its own that imagines and creates by the power of imagination. If man's imagination is strong enough to penetrate into every corner of his interior world, it will be able to create things in those corners, and whatever man thinks will take form in his soul, ... He who wants to know how a man can unite his power of imagination with the power of the imagination of heaven must know by what process this may be done. A man may come into possession of creative power by identifying his own mind with the Universal Mind, and he who succeeds in doing so will be in possession of the highest possible wisdom; the lower realm of nature will be subject to him, and the powers of heaven will aid him, because heaven is the servant of wisdom" . . . "The exercise of true magic does not require any ceremonies or conjurations, or the making of circles or signs; it requires neither benedictions or maledictions, ceremonies or conjurations, neither verbal blessings nor curses; it only requires a strong faith in the omnipotent power of all good, that can accomplish everything if it acts through a human mind who is in harmony with it, and without which nothing useful can be accomplished" . . . "Man is created with great powers; he is greater than heaven and greater than the earth"... "By faith, imagination and will we may accomplish whatever we desire".

Yet, unlike the disciples of schools and systems of medicine, and even his far-away-off followers, the healers of various denominations of our day, Paracelsus in his practice employed whatever mode of cure promised the best results, whether it were a drug or the power of the Holy Ghost. " Ills of the body", he said, "may be cured by physical remedies, or by the power of the Spirit (Holy Ghost ; trance healing) acting through the soul". ... He who possesses the power to cure diseases and to drive out evil influences by the power of the Spirit is ordained of God". Yet, while believing himself to be so ordained, he was at the same time indefatigable in the use of his gift of sensing the presence of medicinal virtues to discover new remedies in whatever substance nature had hid them, and making his discoveries known.

If strict yoga practice was necessary to qualify for all this, a born yogi like him, the opportunity to both learn and pursue it, was afforded by his sojourn of many years in Asiatic countries, and he was not the man to neglect such an opportunity. Many of his ideas are plainly Hindu, and it is highly probable that he traveled and studied in Hindustan. But he was a yogi of his own sort; unlike the Hindu sages, who disregard all magical gifts that come in their way on the yoga path, he appropriated and used them, while, unlike European magicians, he made no secret of them or of the way of acquiring them, save in special cases. Concerning heaven he says: "If we speak of heaven, we then speak of our home, of our own country".

Of the nature of man we have this: "The essential man is not limited by the visible physical form of his material body; his spiritual substance extends as far as the stars. His true self is the spirit of God".

"Before his fall man could rule over the sun and the stars. Everything was in his power. Fire, air, water and earth could not tame him; no fire burned him, no water drowned, no air suffocated him". "No heat, no cold, no sickness, no accident, nor any fear could touch or terrify him. His body could pass through earth and rocks without breaking anything in them; for a man who could be overpowered by the terrestrial nature, or who could be broken to pieces would not be eternal". Here seem to be all the requisites for the terrestrial immortal man which some think will yet enjoy his eternity in physical form on this same material planet. Finally we have : "The soul in the power of God penetrates through all things and is as powerful as God himself", which recalls the "I am Brahman", of the Hindu perfected saint. Where the philosophy of Paracelsus agrees with that of the Hindus he must be presumed to have obtained it from them, and so when we find Boehme, who came long after Paracelsus, giving out as his own the ideas of the latter, he must be considered as his disciple rather than his rival, even when they came to him while in his ecstatic state, and, as he believed, from the Holy Spirit, for it is the well-known habit of inspirations to embody and adapt themselves to the preconceived notions of the mediums through which they come. By the time Boehme appeared the teachings of the other must have got well abroad and ready to be imbibed, even by those who did not read his books. The points of agreement in the doctrines of the two were : The unity of God ; the omnipotence of man; the union, if not identity, of both; the disregard of the personal Jehovah and the historical Jesus, and the resolving of all deity into an impersonal principle; magic as the creative and operative force in Nature. All which was old Hinduism, newly taught, but the new teaching had most important effects on the European minds. It was a protest at once against Protestantism and Romanism, so far as it related to religious notions, and as regards science was a revival of the longneglected methods of the earlier students of Nature as she is, and not as philosophers think she should be.

Boehme

Notwithstanding Luther's effort to stamp out mysticism, there arose in Germany a century after him Jacob Boehme, a believer in miracles, a worker of miracles and a miracle himself. He, too, was, in Hindu parlance, a born yogi. The measure of solitude and leisure possible to him while serving as a herdboy and afterwards while working at the very quiet and lonely trade of shoemaker, sufficed to develop him while as yet a youth into what John of the Cross would have termed a proficient and the Hindus a well advanced candidate, A brief sketch of his mystical experiences and a statement of a few of the leading philosophical ideas which resulted from them will give some idea of the quality of this greatest yogi of Protestant times.

At the age of nineteen Boehme got married, and it was as the head of a family and while working for its support that he did his meditation and contemplation, and got his ecstasies and illuminations, thereby proving that for some natures at least renunciation of the duties of life is not essential to progress in sanctification. But incidents related of him show that he knew the value of solitude, and kept much by himself, and in his " Dialogue between a Scholar or Disciple and His Master" he says: "When thou art ' quiet or silent, then thou art that which God was,'" etc. His methods of concentration were those usual with devotees. An access of the horrors gave rise to devotional concentration, which took form as an intense longing to find the heart of Jesus Christ wherein he might hide himself and find protection from the fearful wrath of God. The result he thus describes:

"While engaged in such an earnest seeking and desiring the door was opened to me, so that in one quarter of an hour I saw and learned more than if I had studied many years in the universities". But a late experience taught him that it mattered not what he concentrated on, for a glittering point in a newly brightened pewter platter that caught his eye and held it for a while sent him into as good an ecstasy as could be wished.

After declaring that, he wrote "only for those who desire to be sanctified and united with the Supreme Power from which they have originated", he gives the following instructions:

"Thine own hearing, willing and seeing prevents thee from seeing God. But if you keep quiet and desist from thinking and feeling within your personal self-hood, then will the eternal hearing, seeing and speaking become revealed to you". "We should be blind and deaf and mute, and know nothing, and know of no life of our own. The practicer "should leave money and goods, father and mother, brother and sister, wife and child, body and life, and his own self should become as nothing to him. He must surrender everything, and become poorer than a bird of the air that has no nest".

But this was only a sub modo renunciation. Having surrendered all his possessions to God, the surrenderer might still hold them of Him as a kind of fief; and thus renunciation be made easy. Boehme wrote his books, as he affirms, under inspirational impression. "I, in my human self, do not know", he said, "what I shall have to write; but whatever I am writing the Spirit dictates to me what to write, and shows me all in such a wonderful clearness that I do not know whether or not I am with my consciousness in this world" . . .

"I might sometimes perhaps write more elegantly and in better style, but the fire burning in me is driving me on. My hand and my pen must then seek to follow the thoughts as well as they can. The inspiration comes like a shower of rain. That which I catch I have. If it were possible to grasp all that I perceive, then would my writings be more explicit". And certainly a reader can readily believe him when he says that it was only while the Holy Ghost was present with him that he himself could understand them. His idea of God is that, " in his primitive aspect he is not to be conceived of as a being, but merely as the power or the intelligence constituting the potentiality for being — as an unfathomable eternal will, wherein everything is contained, and which, although itself everything, is, nevertheless, only one, but desirous of revealing itself and to enter into a state of spiritual being" . . . "God is eternal unity, the unmeasurable one good, having nothing before or after it that could possibly endow it with something or move it. It is, without any inclinations or qualities, without any beginning in time, within itself, only One. This God creates by the exercise of "the divine magic power", which is "the spirit desirous for being. It is essentially nothing but will, but it enters into existence. It is the greatest mystery; it is above nature, and forces nature to assume forms according to the form of its will. It introduces the foundation into the abyss of the groundlessness and changes nothing into something".

CHAPTER XXVI - YOGA IN GENERAL

Methods of Practice

The materials for a comparative study of yoga, so far as I have been able to collect them, are now before the reader. Those which relate to Hindu Yoga are seen to be the most complete of all, and by their sufficiency to make up for the scantiness of the others. It will be observed that the postures, breathings and movements are peculiar to that yoga, and that of these the movements are peculiar to Hatha Yoga, while the postures and breathings, though more or less borrowed from it by the others, have nowhere the prominence accorded to them by the Hatha, being by some prescribed as a preparative practice good for beginners only, and by others merely tolerated as fortifying the health, whereas the Hatha, as set forth by Swatmaram, seems to insist on the importance, if not the necessity, of all its methods. But if the postures, breathings and movements were essential to success, they would be found in all yogas. And this consideration would move us to dismiss them as of inferior importance, were it not that the American experiences, that have before been stated, seem to prove a necessary and wonderful connection to exist between the bodily manifestations on the one part and mental concentration on the other. Those experiences, it will be remembered, showed that mere concentration, unalloyed by any philosophical, ethical or religious admixture, will suffice, if long enough persisted in, to set up, independently of the will of the practicer, all the bodily processes of Swatmaram's book, save only a few that, from their nature, require the concurrence of the conscious will, and that, except the hundred or more movements that were of the nature of mesmeric passes or massage manipulations, those experiences did not go beyond that book. Thus there were brought into play intelligence, force and will — and why not providence also? — from a source beyond the consciousness of the practicer, yet all operating within his body. It is not strange that mankind have generally believed that such manifestations indicate bodily possession by some departed soul or other supernatural being, but those of the present time who study the experiences in question will probably discard that supposition along with the Hindu one of a deva descending from heaven to act as guru, and the Christian one of direct guidance by God's own hand, in favor of the more rational one, as it seems to me, that when a practicer has by his own efforts made a certain progress along the path, nature comes to his aid and conducts him the rest of the way. Whether all practicers may expect to be thus favored, that is to say, whether all men are so constituted as to be thus acted on is another question. Probably all of us have, in some degree, magical capabilities, whether for developing or operative magic, by which I mean that all are possible prophets. Probably all, whether in any measure or in no measure at all developed as such, may do prophet's work by prophet's methods, i.e. by force of thought, will, or whatever other force comes at the prophet's call. That he has spirits, genii or gods in waiting we may well doubt, but that there are natural forces which, if rightly invoked, will do his bidding may not be doubted. It is to be noted that the American experiences reproduced Hatha Yoga and no other. So far from sustaining the claim of the mental yogists that Hatha is at best but a preparation for entering on the practice of their methods, those experiences show that it is just their methods that can inaugurate it. And the teachings of Swatmaram, though giving no precedence to concentration, make it and the physical exercise go along together, the two combining to form a complete yoga system of dignity and importance and sufficiency too great for it to be put to use as a mere preparatory discipline, whether its value as such be, as some say, to strengthen the body, or as others say, to give a sort of initial control over the mind, in aid of its studies in discriminative philosophy, etc, The school of Sankaracharya, which chiefly controls modern Hindu thought, gives as a reason for making Hatha practice merely subservient to its own, that by the former only a temporary release from re-births can be obtained, which release will come to an end with the destruction of the presently existing universe, whereas the latter ensures an eternal release. But we of the West do not yet know that there is any re-birth to be feared, nor that yoga practice would give release from it if there were. Both alike lie beyond the powers of perception and the forms of knowing we are accustomed to rely on.

A better reason for preferring mental yoga to physical is to be found enveloped in Sankaracharya's allusion in the Vedant Sara, before quoted, to the severe mortifications of former yogis, which were such as in his time mankind were no longer capable of enduring. Doubtless the former yogis of the valley of the Indus were better able to undergo austerities than the later ones of the valley of the Ganges, but the enervating effects of a torrid climate would better excuse the deterioration that followed the abandonment by the Hindu race of its northern home, which is indicated by the saying of one authority that a really great yogi is now "the rare efflorescence of a century", than justify a preference for the easier practice as being in itself better than the harder. Like the magicians of the Indus, those of the Akkadian highlands probably lost quality after their emigration into the hot plains of Babylonia, and thereby ultimately lost control of the vast empire whose civilization they created there. Perhaps, too, in some remote age the Hindus and Akkadians were one race, with one magic, and that magic Hatha Yoga.

As it is to-day, Hindu Yoga stands distinguished from all others by this, that it has two supports, namely, mental stillness and bodily movement, thus combining intellectual and physical training, while those others have only the first, obtainable by concentration or its equivalents, in the shape of religious devotion, etc., which operate by virtue of the concentration they involve. It must be admitted that the best method of developing man should include the whole of him, and since Hatha Yoga includes more of him than the others do, its superiority to them must follow. Besides this, it is the purest magic of them all, having had its origin in simple times before philosophy or religion came to trouble it, and when only worldly welfare was cared for; and since the needs of every-day life are more urgent than those of any future one, the resort to magic must in those times have been extensive and habitual to a degree quite unknown in these. In fact, and to speak plainly, the task of the student of magic in this century consists mainly in digging through the rubbish of religion and philosophy which, during fifty or a hundred former ones, have been heaped upon it.

First to be considered, in entering upon our study, are the conditions proper to yoga practice; secondly, the various methods of it; thirdly, the results obtainable; and, fourthly, the object and aim of it held in view in each system.

Conditions

Solitude. Although none of the systems of yoga treats social life as absolutely inconsistent with successful practice, yet all of them regard it as a serious hindrance, and, as a rule, yogis have been solitaries or recluses whenever they could. Neither Zoroaster in his cave, Buddha beneath his bo tree, Moses on Sinai, Jesus on the Mount of Olives, nor Mohammed in his grotto, had anybody to keep him company there. And the presence of supernatural intruders, in the shape of gods and saints, devils and demons, such as the practicer's own imagination objectifies when he reaches the stage of visions and voices, is no more desirable than the presence of real persons would be, since they equally break the spell of his solitude. He should, in fact, aim to have no social existence at all. His business is with himself and nobody else. Not all the world could help him with it save by keeping away from him. Alone in the matrix he began the making of himself, and alone he can best continue that process. Ethics are for the social man and not for him. Love and sympathy, hate and antipathy, are disturbing emotions which, if allowed play, would make all his practice vain. Care for the well-being of family or neighborhood is utterly inconsistent with his entirely selfish undertaking of getting to his very self, all by himself.

Silence. The Chinese sage of old Taoism, we are told, " shut his mouth and made his instructions consist in silence". In monastic communities silence in a measure serves as a substitute for solitude, keeping the members mentally apart though bodily congregated. In this the Trappists go far beyond the other Christian orders, but all of them practice sitting mute as a mode of discipline and worship; it is a condition of yoga practice with the Buddhists and Mohammedans as well.

Poverty. Though Christian asceticism seems to prize poverty as being not merely a condition in aid of quietude, but also as a form of penitential misery, its real value to the yogi lies in the detachment it effects from worldly interests. A substitute for it is moral detachment, or a mental habit of not caring for wealth, or any of the enjoyments it brings, by force of which the practicer is made to live and act, feel and think just as he would if actually a beggar, which, according to Jacob Boehme and some others, is as good as being one, though the better opinion is that for him who tramps the yoga path real beggary is a surer means than any imitation of it, for getting left alone.

Detachment, as has been seen, is much insisted on in those works on yoga that give details concerning methods. It signifies renunciation, not merely of earthly goods, but of whatever can attach to earthly life. Complete detachment in fact constitutes that state of equanimity to reach which, according to Boethius, " one must drive away joy and hope and grief and fear"; and which when attained, according to Plotinus, exempts from all the pangs of sympathy. It was the principle of stoicism, and appears to have incarnated in the peaceable but lawless, good but godless, Eskimo race.

Disagreeable surroundings have been considered proper conditions by Christian ascetics, but not by Hindu Yogis, whose manuals recommend comfortable homes with pleasant scenery, and who when they practice, instead of the kneeling posture of a slave, take the easier and more dignified one proper for him who in his own home awaits to receive as his equal the God of the Universe.

Methods

First and before all others is concentration. Solitude, silence, poverty and detachment, have their value only in so far as they are favoring conditions to concentration, the meaning and importance of which have been so often set forth in what has been cited from the teachings of those sages who left us full expositions of their methods, and implied in what we otherwise know of those who did not, that no further explanation of them is needed now. In some of the quotations the words "meditation" and "contemplation" are made to stand for concentration in a way that is confusing. Both mean concentration, but properly applied each means a different stage of it; at least so John of the Cross, Molinos and Guillaume Postel define them. But it is well to repeat here, what the quotations abundantly prove, that it is the concentration that does the work and not the thing concentrated on. All attempts to teach either philosophy or religion by means of yoga are attempts to pervert it, whether the point held up for the mind to fix itself on be, as Sankafacharya recommends, "This is not me", or as Postel suggests, "The infinite wickedness of man". To set out on the path with expectation that it will conduct you to absolute truth, and that that truth is formulated in the Sankhya philosophy, which you are already instructed in so far as mere instruction can go, is to ensure that at the end a "spiritual impression" will confirm both preconceptions, and that what you begun by believing in with your outer reason you will end by knowing, or "realizing", as it is called, with your inmost sense of knowledge — or feeling sure you do so. Yoga thus prac ticed may yield all other yoga results, but it will be with the disturbing addition of a fixed belief, proved in no better way than the fixed beliefs of visionaries usually are.

" All life is thought, all beings are contemplations" said Plotinus; and again, "Since Nature is not an action, she is a contemplation". The Greeks practiced concentration in the Eleusinian mysteries, and believed that by it a soul could redeem itself from hades. The Buddhists say of their creative God: "From his tapas (meditation) the universe was produced by him". An ancient Chinese author boasts of his people's superior "power of concentration"; and everywhere in the literature of old magic we come upon the word or its equivalent, as expressing both the method of the gods in creating and ruling the world and those of men developing themselves as magicians, and as such rivalling those same gods in doing work of like sort with theirs. When, a few years ago, magical healing under its various names made its appearance in America, I found it easier to believe in its good results than to understand its methods, even after reading a large bookful of expositions of them and taking four courses of lessons from different instructors. Each of these taught that it was the recognition of certain truths by the patient as well as the healer that effected the cure — but this only on condition that those truths were understood and realized. I do not think that any sick or well person was ever able to do this, yet still the healing went on. A year of speculation brought me to the conclusion that a certain mental attitude, such as the thinking out of abstruse problems or trying to think out incomprehensible ones involves, tended to induce in the thinker a magical healing power. Here I rested during, perhaps, another year, but at length was able to take one step further, and decide that the attitude in question consisted in the arrestation of thought. Years later I was confirmed in this by consulting Hindu works on yoga. But how does stopping his thinking make a yoga of a man?

As all know, every thought is an expenditure of the mysterious force whose inflow, whether from a spiritual or material source it matters not, constitutes human life. And when we consider how small an expenditure of thought is really needed to carry an ordinary mortal through his daily duties, and yet, what a constant stream of it runs through his head from dawn to dark, we see that an enormous waste of life is the ordinary attendant on living.

The same force that first produced a given man, and has since sustained him in being, for some reason continues to superabundantly flow into him, the superabundance, like the overflow of a mill-dam, running out of him as continuously in, for the most part, useless ideation. Concentration, in such measure as it saves this waste by stopping the thinking, places at the disposal of Nature for whatever other work on the man she has in hand, making a yogi of him, for instance, an extra supply of force; thus, to arrest thought is to accumulate force.

The Breathings

Breathing gives activity to the mind by supplying arterialized blood to its organ, the brain, and holding the breath, by diminishing that supply retards thinking, thus accomplishing by physical restraint what in concentration is accomplished by moral restraint, namely, the saving up of vital force by curtailing its expenditure in thought. All the three modes of breath restraint that have been described show by their effects that nature puts this saved-up force to use by producing within the body in the first instance, and for some ulterior purpose which need not now be considered, certain vibrations, tensions and other movements of the same sort as mental concentration produces, but the method that consists in quite emptying the lungs, and holding them empty as long as may be, so that the smallest possible supply of arterialized blood reaches the brain, produces those movements in a more marked degree than do the other two, one of which consists in holding in the lungs all the air they can be made to receive and the other in retaining whatever quantity happens to be there when the breathing begins, indicating that the more absolute the exclusion of air is, the more so is the arrest of thought, if we may measure that arrest by the movements into which the saved force is diverted. This holding out, will very often, make the whole body shake or sweat, or both. But the other two methods go further than suppress thought ; they introduce into the body whatever elements of vitality accompany the inflowing atmosphere — whatever of cosmic force from without is pressing to come in and thereby convert itself into vital force, opening to this an access additional to what the surface of the body affords. Ordinary breathing does the same, it is true, but these yoga breathings give nature more time than it does to appropriate the influx by ten to one. In performing them there will be felt a peculiar tensive fullness of the whole body reaching to the nails of the fingers and toes and even the roots of the teeth. Says Chuang-Tzü, in his only allusion to the breathings, and which is too brief to qualify the statement before made, that they are not included in any other than Hindu Yoga: "Pure men draw breath from their heels" — an expression that recalls one of Swatmaram's sutras, which reads: "He should practice Kumbhaka until he feels that prana pervades the whole of his body from the head to the toe". Whatever may be the nature of the elements of life that from without enter the human body, and whether they be many or one, it has always been believed that something so enters, and pervades that organism. This something has furnished much material for speculation. The Chinese give it the all-inclusive name of Tao, the Hindus call it Prana, or life-breath, and in modern science it goes incognito as vital force. But here the question will naturally arise: Why do not the ordinary ten breaths a minute let in as much or more of the vital force as one long-drawn breath retained for a whole minute? The ordinary breathing, short and frequent, certainly suffices to supply the blood with oxygen. Why not also to supply the organism with whatever else it wants that comes in with that oxygen? But there is a difference between ten quick taps and one slow pressure, between ten short vibrations and one long one, difference enough to make of one thing quite another thing, both as to action and effect. Whoever tries them will know that the yoga breaths do in fact produce effects which ordinary ones do not, and be apt to presume that this is because the long ones give more time than the short ones do for the inflowing force to act, as imparting, and the organism, as receiver, to appropriate. The beneficial effects of the yoga breathings seem evident enough, and there is no a priori reason why they should not be what they seem. The Hindus carry their belief in it so far as in certain cases to blow into the bladder through a kind of catheter. Just as the body of him who bathes in the ocean has the benefit of every medicament water can dissolve and it receive, the same body has the benefit of every force of nature that can come in with the breath, and remain long enough to be taken up.

Sound. In connection with the breathings certain sounds are directed to be made, namely, by " putting the tongue between the lips and drawing the breath in the mouth with a hissing sound " — by — "protruding the tongue a little way beyond the lips and then inhaling" — by "filling in the air rapidly, making the sound of a male bee, and again exhaling it make the sound of a female bee humming".

One effect of making these sounds in the way described is, of course, the retardation of the inflow or outflow of the breath, and so of the thinking process, but we are led to look for a directly exerted magical action of the sounds themselves as such, when we consider how important a part music has played in ancient magic, and this notwithstanding that in the synopsis that has been given of Hindu Yoga, all said about musical sounds is comprised in what has just been quoted, in what is found in the directions for practicing Laya Yoga, and in Sabhatapy's directions that in making its divine pilgrimage through the body, the mind should at certain points sing a "mantram" to the spirit there ruling. The priests of Egypt insisted on the utmost exactness in the temple chants. The Hebrew prophet Elisha called for music to tune his soul to prophesy. David with his harp charmed away the evil spirit sent by Jehovah to afflict Saul. Plato, when he describes the four manias or ecstatic states "by which the soul could be led back to its pristine felicity", gives the musical mania the first place. Turning to Akkadian magic we find that though concentration is implied in the fact that magical powers were acquired, yet that when these powers were put in operation it was nearly always by means of incantation. The Kalevala shows that the Finnic gods and magicians alike did their work chiefly by singing. The gnostics worked, says Plotinus, "by enchantment, charms, cries, aspirations, whistling", — but to return to Hindu methods:

The Laya Yoga consists wholly in listening to certain sounds that can be heard within the practicer's body when the ears are closed, and which are collectively termed "The Nâda". " In the beginning they resemble those of the ocean, the clouds, the kettle-drum, and zazara (a sort of drumcymbal) ; in the middle those arising from the mardala, the conch, the bell and the horn. In the end those of the tinkling bells, the flutes, the vina and the bees. Thus are heard the various sounds from the middle of the body". The results of this Laya practice are very prompt in coming, according to Swatmaram, who says that "Great yogis who practice Samadhi through concentration on Nâda, experience a joy in their hearts that surpasses all description". Certainly the American experiences tend to prove that the sounds produced in breathing have power over the bodily sensations, aside from the part they play in restraining the outgoing breath. They seem to bring the bodily vibrations into unison with themselves and also to strengthen them. The American sounds answer very well to the description just given of the Nâda.

Dancing is in all magic except Christian. Both it and music are well adapted to what may be termed congregational practice, where many take part. To be sure. King David was not a pretty sight when he performed before the Ark, anymore than a row of shaking Quakers are, but none will deny that such ballet troupes as have in all times been attached to pagan temples must have " drawn " with a force not to be despised. When Wesley introduced lively tunes into Methodist worship, he said it was because he saw no reason for letting Satan have all the good music. Wesley's innovation is extending, but as yet no movement has been made to appropriate for the service of the Christian sanctuary the allurement that lies in beautiful form in graceful movement, and these still remain the monopoly of the Christian devil and heathen gods.

Devotion. Intense religious anxiety, glad religious hopes and loving yearnings cultivated in every Christian church compel concentration of mind. But the humdrum litanies, droning chants, and soporific incense, the tiresome genuflexions, bead-telling, repetition of aves and paters, the fixing of the gaze on the crucifix, turning of the eyes upward just as in Hindu yoga practice, and long and short retreats, such as the Church of Rome has devised, prove that better than the others she knows the value of magic as a support to faith.

Fasting is commonly thought to help the ascetic to be chaste, by weakening his body and thereby its passions, but it is hard to see the advantage of rousing up one violent craving, which hunger is, to put down another no more violent, nor how, since yoga consists in perfecting the man in all his parts, fasting severe enough to impair health can be deemed good practice. Yet occasional fasts, for special purposes, undergone by yogis in good condition, may be supposed to accumulate

power just as arresting thought or breath does. The ever-flowing current of the life breath, relieved of the labor of digesting food, is set free for yoga uses. So, too, with Vigils. The Christian monastic leaves his bed and begins his vigil about two o'clock in the morning; so does the Hindu, according to "The Science of Breath". Now that is the time when the labor of digestion having been accomplished. Nature employs her forces in doing her plastic work, that is to say, in converting the fluids she has been producing from the food into solid tissues of the body. But this can only be done while it is sleeping, and so it is that by waking it at the time in question and holding it so the vital force is saved that would otherwise be spent in body building, which is postponed until the vigil is ended. For other reasons midnight is the most propitious time for concentration. It is then that the body is most at rest, and solitude and silence bathe the watcher in quietude.

Tiresome repetitions, whether devotional or not, is good practice. And in the number of these imposed on the Hindu Yogi the Romish ritual is far outgone. Certain French savants of the present time who have waded into magic as far as what, to hide their shame, they have named hypnotism, have found out the value of tiresome repetition, and one of them has invented a mechanical means to it in the shape of a whirligig, which, being intently looked at as it whirls, brings on the hypnotic state, by fatiguing the looker's eyes, as is supposed. The tiresome method, instead of restraining the wasteful flow of thought as concentration does, by holding the mind still, puts it to sleep. Stupefaction which falls short of sleep is considered a good result and to indicate hopeful progress on the path, no less by Hindu Swatmaram's commentator than by Spanish John of the Cross; and both give warning that it will increase till it reaches a stage wherein the yogi becomes incapable of taking care of himself, or performing the necessary duties of life without guidance, which the Hindu says may be afforded by another man, but, according to the Christian, is given in a miraculous way by God himself, as before stated, and there can be no doubt but that the moderate doles of it allowed by the Catholic Church to its children is wholesome and comforting, and being by the children supposed to come from the breast of their spiritual mother, helps confirm their faith in her teachings, just as the whirling crescent or cluster of mirrors arouses the faith of Dr. Luy's patients in the truth of his suggestions while lulling them to quietude and slumber. Swatmaram commends the practice of the murcha Kumbhalca for the reason that, as he says: "It reduces the mind to a state of stupor and gives pleasure".

Spells. The reliance which has been had in all systems of magic on the one word spell, such as the Egyptian "Ammon", the Jewish "Jah-Veh" and the Hindu "Om" is hard to comprehend. Yet so important was it esteemed by the founders of Christianity that the new religion should not be behind the old ones in this respect that they incarnated a spell referred to as "the word", and put it into their Trinity. Longer formulas, such as adjurations to depart addressed to the devil, and longer still, such as were the incantations of Egyptian and Chaldean magic, or the philosophical statements which Christian scientists and other modern healers address to their patients may work by way of concentration or suggestion, or by force of their logic or tiresomeness, but this would not account for any single word, even though it be the name of a god, having magical power, or the reputation of it. Yet wonderful stories are told by Hindus of the potency of their word Om., the "Yoga Vasishtha", devoting fifty pages to it, and conjuring with names has always been common with magicians of all degrees, whether priestly or lay.

Celibacy. Notwithstanding the exceptions heretofore noted, there can be no doubt that absolute chastity has always been considered a better method than deviation from it to any degree, and in most systems, as shown by the quotations heretofore given, has been rigorously insisted on. The Christian Church may have had many good reasons for imposing celibacy on her priesthood, but none could have been more cogent than its value, made known by the experiences of the monks of the desert and cloister, as a condition to magical practice. Not only is the existence of a family inconsistent with solitude, silence, inaction and quietude, but the calling one into existence involves a drain on vital force, that is, on magical force. The chastity of the yogi is better named diversion than suppression, and to resort to mutilation, as the Bible says some have done for the Kingdom of Heaven's sake, would be exceeding bad practice, and the fact that no yoga scripture that has been quoted names or sanctions it tends to prove that, in the judgment of the wise authors of them, the organs concerned have functions to perform even in the organism of a celibate. Of course, emasculation would save a deal of selfrestraint, and, of course, without it there will be a disturbance ; for years the practicer may have to battle with beautiful devils, as Saint Anthony did, but, soon or late, the yogis say, the compensation will come, and all will be peace.

Penance. Self-torment as a magical method must be in some way efficacious, for it has place in all systems, the Christian Church, as I have said, putting it to the additional use of forestalling punishment for sin. Apuleius, who wrote in the second century A.D., in his "Golden Ass" describes a scourging, which for a very base, but yet purely magical purpose, a devotee of Isis gave himself thus: "Seizing, therefore, a whip, which it is usual for these half men to carry with them, and which consisted of twisted woolen fillets, hanging down in long fringes, and is chequered with many pastern joints of sheep, he gave himself with it many lashes, which were severe on account of the numerous knots of the whip, being fortified with wonderful firmness against the pain of the blows". This man and his companions, who went through other like performances, and whom Apuleius termed "filthy catamites", wound up with a feast procured with the pence flung at them by the attendant crowd, which closed in a disgusting orgy. The Christian flagellants, so numerous in the thirteenth, fourteenth and fifteenth centuries, though following the pagan method, set up for themselves as object the very opposite result of maintaining their chastity by mortifying the flesh, but, strange as it may seem, these pious persons, who also went about the country whipping themselves on their bare haunches for the edification of the crowd, arrived in so many cases at a very pagan result that the Church, which had at first favored the movement as being in the interest of religion, had to take measures to arrest it. It has by no means died out, however, nor ceased to be honored and encouraged by the applause of that very large body of good Catholics who, like the throng that followed the flagellating Greek catamites, are able to enjoy the sufferings of other people. Scene, the city of Philadelphia; time, the culmination of the nineteenth century. The late Catholic bishop of that city, the already beati fied John Neuman, destined in due time to be Saint John, namesake and imitator of him of the Cross, was accustomed to whip himself, it is said, in true flagellant fashion. His scourge, it is true, had but one lash, but the principle of it was the same as that of those used by the catamite Apuleius mentions, being long and weighted at the end, so that it could be wielded over the shoulder and made to reach the objective point of attack, and having a sharp nail at the end, which made a Russian knout of it, was really a severer instrument than the woolen cat-o'-nine-tails of the pagan flagellants. Our John of Philadelphia seems to have been a close follower of John of the Cross in other respects. He not only wore the same kind of barbed girdle that the other did, but had the same disposition to selfabasement. He slept on a plank, kept himself poor by giving away whatever he had to give, and, when notified by his Archbishop that he was to be made bishop, fell on his knees and with tears in his eyes begged the latter not to appoint one so unworthy as himself. Like his exemplar, too, he ruined his health and shortened his life by austerities.

CHAPTER XXVII - RESULTS OF PRACTICE AND INDICATIONS OF PROGRESS

Vibrations

The conditions being given and the methods practiced, the first effects perceived, so far as the American experiences have made known the order of their coming, are vibrations, resembling those of an electric or magnetic current, which, unless mentally directed elsewhere, begin in the feet and thence mount by gradations upward and spread over the whole body, tarrying on the way at each of the great nerve-centres and reaching at last a point at the top of the head, called by the Hindus the Brahmandra, occupying in their course a measure of time varying from a few days to many years, according to the receptivity and diligence of the practicer. At first amounting to merely a gentle prickling of the surface, these vibrations attain to different degrees of fineness and emphasis, steadily increasing in force and pleasantness from the time when they start to ascend from the feet upward, with sensations a Hindu book describes as of — "Brahman creeping up the legs", until they invade the profundity of the nerves and thrill the whole organism with what John of the Cross calls " touches of God" and describes as being so sweet that only one of them would compensate for a lifetime of woe. This to the beginner is a far-off result, but once the earliest prickling is felt, he may be sure the "current of the life-breath" has been turned on, and that from thence onward, conditions being maintained and practice kept up, will continually labor to carry him forward toward yoga. Out of the vibrations come certain tonic pressures and tensions, and out of them, in seemingly well-ordered sequence, the whole train of phenomena between here and there, extending even unto ultimate Samadhi.

The first and usually the very prompt results after the vibrations begin, especially if these are aided by the breathings, are improved health and strength, showing forth in a more symmetrical shape, a more graceful carriage, a smoother and livelier skin, often puffed out, as it were, and tinged with a rosy hue, more expressive and brighter eyes, and sometime a partial restoration of gray hair to its original color, or elfacement of wrinkles. Withal, the appetite for food is diminished and the senses sharpened. Following in the train of these, the yoga literature, especially that of primitive times, promises, and with emphasis, shall come other signs of rejuvenescence, a promise which some American experiences are thought to justify, as also those may which have already been told concerning Postel, who, if he is to be believed, saw a woman of fifty and upwards, look fifteen, and if his contemporaries are to be believed, after he had got to be old, gray and wrinkled, was well started on his way backward toward his youth when the Church laid her hand on him. It cannot be without some foundation that beliefs have always prevailed in the possibility of an indefinitely long extension of earthly life, and even theories, dreams and hopes of earthly immortality. For instance, Lao-Tsee claimed to have lived a thousand years, and his disciple, Chuang-Tzü called himself two hundred older. The Cumaean Sibyl was supposed to have been a thousand years old when she died, or disappeared. Roger Bacon claimed that alchemy "could prolong life to several centuries". The Bible gives the ages of the antediluvian patriarchs in numbers less round than these, but more plausible. And the many great Hindu Siddhas, of whom Swatmaram names thirty-six, who, as he says, "still live and move about the world", if his words be true of them at the present time, must be set down as immortal enough for all present purposes.

As he goes on, each of the practicer's senses will be visited by objectified subjective experiences, nowise less vivid than if supported by objective realities. He will see lights, colors and forms, hear speech and music, smell odors, taste food and touch and feel touches. Nature has taken control of the channels of his senses, and he is subject to revelations, which, according to his preconceptions, will come from gods or saints, demons or devils — in receiving which, however, as John of the Cross seems to have found out, he is only talking to himself. Here is where religions are made and repaired. In America we are not without proof in confirmation of what the history of mysticism in other countries contains respecting these illusions. On the contrary, there is an embarrassing richness of demonstration that as illusions they are realities. One person whom I know is haunted with an odor of violets, another is entertained with exquisite music, etc., and vocal messages seem getting to be as common and cheap as chips.

Much less common, but still common enough to prove themselves, and here and now, too, are such purely physical and objective effects as the levitation of the practicer's body, the exhalation from it of agreeable odors and the radiation from it of lights. The comparatively recent floating in and out of the window of Home, better authenticated than the ascent to the sky of Elijah, or the lifting up to the ceiling of John of the Cross and Theresa, helps us to believe in the possibility of overcoming gravitation, as, indeed, should every case where a ponderable object is raised so much as an inch from its position. But for one dollar admittance persons and things can now be seen hanging as high in the air as the monk and nun did. In like manner the stories of the "odor of sanctity", said to have been so pungent about the disinterred body of the same monk as to have identified it nine months after burial, and to have emanated from the living bodies of many other saints, are rendered credible by the accounts we have of the same kind of manifestations occurring now, and illuminated features and rings of light like those which crown the idols of the Virgin Mary and the Japanese "Queen of Heaven", and other divinities of earlier date than either, have of late become so familiar as to justify belief that they were founded on fact, as also the account we have of the transfiguration on Mount Tabor, where the face of Jesus " shone like the sun and his garments became white as light". All these phenomena must be expected to occur as effects of yoga practice if long enough continued.

What has been said in the account heretofore given of the American experiences concerning the movements, namely, that at each recurrence of them the same serial order was observed as that by which one by one they originally arose, may also be affirmed of the vibrations and other sensations, such as those of pressure and tension. At least a habit of Nature to go back to the beginning each time she resumes her left-off work, as if to get her hand in, and at the same time hold on to progress already gained, is indicated by some experiences that have come under my observation, and which recall what Haeckel says in his "Evolution of Man" concerning Nature's mode of working the series of transformations undergone by the foetus in the womb, in which we have "a complete picture of the remarkable series of forms through which the animal ancestors of the human race have passed from the beginning of organic creation to the first appearance of man". Thus, for instance, a pressure first felt on the nerve-centre at the ankle, and that after being felt there and only there for months, ascended to the nerve-centre at the knee, whence, after tarrying, perhaps, as long, it went up to the groins, and so on till the top of the head was reached, will, in most every instance, begin its course at the ankle each time any part above there is to be touched.

The activities set up in the practicer's organism, in due time become more or less habitual, or automatic, and probably also unconscious; the recognition of which by Christian mystical writers is found in their use of such terms as "oraison" (orison), "secret meditation", "unconscious meditation", "virtual and acquired contemplation", "habit of union", "habit of internal recollection", "virtual prayer", as if the organism after a while become receptive enough to the new force to admit and react to it as of its own motion — for a time at least — as if meditation originated movements, which afterwards go on of themselves, taking advantage of every moment of mental quietude to do so. For instance, the practicer will, when in a calm state of mind he listens to a conversation, or to music, or reads a book with close attention, feel the vibrations, etc., at their accustomed work, giving him the comfort of knowing he is not losing time (One of the recognized methods of Hindu Yoga practice is Dharana, or

Dhyana which means the steadying of the mind by study). It was a similar manifestation of the uninvoked yoga principle that interrupted the conversation of John of the Cross and Theresa in the convent parlor, and raised them both to the ceiling, and that at another time compelled the monk to grasp the bars of the grating to hold himself down to earth, and made him to fear to let his mind "dwell on anything" lest there should be a scene, and that caused in other pious men sensations and movements so improper as to compel them to pray less often, or not at all. But with the disciples of Molinos, who did not push things so far, such habitual working of the principle in question was all-important, since it enabled them to attend to the ordinary duties of life, and yet make their way towards sanctity. And the beautiful results the Quietists thus obtained should be most encouraging to those who in the agitating conditions that prevail in Christian countries may undertake yoga practice. Thus might be obtained, without seclusion in any cloistered prison or enclosure within any church pale, the development of all the wealth of magical power.

But if it be true, as is commonly thought, that the multitude really desire to be enclosed within some kind of religious pale, then this principle of automatic yoga movement is of great importance, since it renders practicable the embodying of Quietistic magic into the new Christianity which religious experts are now trying to construct out of what is left of the old, a thing that should by all means be done, even if only for weaning purposes.

The exhibition of miracles possible only to a yogi of some degree, and the inner sensations of a comforting kind that yoga practice causes, have been the indispensable supports of every religion that has been able to stand in times past; and religion builders who do not know that it must always be so have not learned their trade. All revelations, true or false, testifying in favor of this or that faith, have been spoken by the mouths, or written by the pens of the prophets, that is, of magicians, and been accepted as true, because the revealers were also wonder workers. Faith, which enables men, if not to move mountains, at least to swallow mountainous incredibilities, is a state of true magical ecstasy just as is the "sweetness of the flesh " which Thomas a Kempis calls it, but others call the love of God, and in fine so are all those pleasant experiences which concentration in prayer can bring to the afflicted, known as religious consolation. It is claimed that even Calvinists can feel this.

Bliss. Into a state of enjoyment worthy of this name the vibrations ultimately run. Rama Pashad says: "And drawn by the taste of bliss (ananda) the mind sets itself to working out with greater and greater zeal the process of its evolution". In Swatmaram's book the practicer is repeatedly encouraged to persevere by the promise of bliss, which is there characterized as "an undefinable joy" ; as " the indescribable state of Laya which can be experienced by the yogi alone". Of two certain Mudras it says: "Though apparently differing in the position of the eyes and places to which the attention or mind is directed, they are one in their result. Both of them bring about a state of bliss". Again it declares that when the mind becomes one with the object concentrated on: "Let there be Mukti or not, here is uninterrupted bliss", and again, "The great yogis who practice Samadhi through the concentration on the Nâda (sounds heard in the body) experience a joy arising in their hearts that surpasses all description". The same joy was referred to by the twelve thousand and more wives of Krishna, when they lauded him for his complaisance to them not withstanding that, being a god, "he had all joy within himself". John of the Cross, in detailing the experiences of spiritual men, says: "Their sense of taste is also deliciously affected; and that of the touch so sweetly caressed at times the bones and marrow exult and rejoice, bathed as it were in joy". The Neoplatonists claimed that by contemplation they arrived at a realization not only of absolute truth, but of absolute blessedness also. Of the witches of much later times it is recorded "They were plunged in vague, unspeakable pleasure" — "They enjoy there a paradise of delight". Nicholas Flamel, the alchemist, says in his book: "The process of the work is very pleasing to nature". That is, to the body. (And another alchemistic work says the students of magic were encouraged to persevere by the bodily pleasure that they derived from it. It should be remembered that the later alchemists declared that their art was a personal development — that the body of the individual was "modified by alchemy", as Roger Bacon, who was one of them, expressed it). And later still, the sect of ecstatics of whom Jane Lead was the historian, enjoyed their meditations so much they were loath to suspend them even at the call of hunger. As further showing that the bliss, blessedness, beatitude in question is a sensuous enjoyment, and comes as ready-payment for daily practice, and not, as some may want to have it, as a mental delight excited by the hope and belief that the deserving soul will some day go to heaven and enjoy bliss there, we have the words of St. Thomas a Kempis, where he advises that the "sweetness of the flesh " be endured rather than enjoyed because it is sweet, in this agreeing with John of the Cross, who says the ascetic must not take any pleasure "in these apprehensions"; that we may prize the love that is in them but not the joy. To the same point I quote from Von Kraft Ebing's " Sexual Psychopathy", the following concerning the experiences of two "heroines of flagellation": "Maria Magdalena, daughter of parents of high position, was a nun of the order of Carmelites, at Florence, in 1580. The flagellations she received, and still more the consequences of that kind of penance, have given her great celebrity and a name in history. Her greatest happiness was when the prioress made her hold her hands behind her back and had her whipped on the naked reins in presence of all the sisters of the convent". Consumed by internal heat and raving always of love, she would cry out when under the lash: "Enough! do not stir any more the fire that devours me. That is not the kind of death I want; there would be too much pleasure in it, too many charms". It is said of the dear lady that "she was often on the point of losing her chastity". Of the other, Elizabeth de Genton, very much the same is related: "The flagellation put her into the delirium of a bacchante. She was seized with a sort of rage when, excited by an extraordinary scourging, she believed herself married to her ideal". This state procured her a happiness so intense that she often cried out: "O love! O infinite love! O love! O creatures, shout then with me: Love! Love!" In both these cases it seems plain that the bliss was as fleshly as the stimulation that produced it. Nevertheless, in the interest of decency and truth, a protest should here be entered against the innuendoes of Boileau and Meibominus, the historians cited as his authorities by Von Kraft Ebing. What the nature of the sensations was that made both ladies rave in terms of human love is not easily to be found out, but they could not have been like those confessed to by the Saints Armelle and Elizabeth, which implied a passion for the infant Jesus and temptations like those of St. Anthony of Padua. The ecstatic states of the fair flagellants lasted for hours, and were experienced in presence of witnesses, as in the case of the nun Magdalena. As for the consuming heat that made St. Catherine of Geneva cry out that she was burning up, it was, doubtless, of the same kind as that felt by King Saul when suddenly developed as a prophet, and that made him fling off his clothes and lie on the ground all night. It was the veritable saintly ardor which ascetics love to feel as a symptom of progress. It is also a troublesome symptom in insane asylums, and was formerly treated by tying on the clothes and binding the hands of the sufferer behind his back, but now by seclusion in a wellwarmed room till it passes off of itself. Physicians say it indicates a peculiar electric state of the skin, and leave us as wise as before, but do not connect it with any blissful state. Another quotation made by Von Kraft Ebing as showing that immodest states may result from devotional ones is a prayer from a very old missal, running thus: "O! that I may have found thee, most charming Emanuel, that I may have thee in my bed! How my soul and my body would rejoice if I had! Come, come to my dwelling, my heart shall be thy chamber!" About as strong language as this we have seen to have been used by Saint John of the Cross in his verses detailing his secret rendez-vous with his beloved. But does either instance prove anything more than that when the vague joy of an occult love craves expression, it has to clothe itself in language of natural love for want of a vocabulary of its own, that language having been in the times in question simpler and honester than now? The obscene formulas of Egyptian worship, the phallic symbols that used to adorn the temples of all old religions, and the dancing women attached to them, must, upon any estimate that can fairly be made of the morality taught there, be so incongruous with it as to force a construction that robs them of any vulgar, literal meaning. But though the strange joy of hidden source that ascetics of all times have gloried in, and which now, perhaps, as much as ever, compensates the inmates of cloisters for all the pleasures of the outer world and all the hardships of internal discipline does not belong to human love, it still belongs to a love, and there is a close enough resemblance between the two evinced by the fact just noticed, that the one takes on the same modes of expressing its ardor as the other, to say nothing of the many other points of resemblance that will presently be mentioned to prove that both have a common root, or, rather, that the one springs from the other, and also prove that both are of the body.

And what is this other love that comes without a lover, that begins with vibrations, conducts to ecstasy and ends in trance ? The Chinese sages named it Tao. The Buddhist, who, contrary to the other Hindus, insist that knowledge does all, contend that love does all, call it simply love. Christians say it is the love of God. The Sufis name it secret or mysterious love. Plato, who declared that it was of itself sufficient to conduct man to perfection, gives it, perhaps, the best name of all — the "Amatory Mania". Let the one love be called, for our purpose here, the higher and the other the lower. In further proof that the love whose thrills made the fair ecstatics rave was not the lower — in other words, that the two are distinct from each other while yet akin — we have the fact that as the higher arises the lower dies out, and while giving birth to it gives place to it. It is known that an unused organ atrophies and becomes merely rudimentary; also that celibacy of itself, if consistently persisted in, will often render a breach of it impossible. But when in connection with it there is yoga practice such as members of the cloistered orders always have enough of for the purpose, the result in question must pretty surely follow. John of the Cross, who knew all about such things, encourages those who may suffer from impure excitement such as has been mentioned, by assuring them that it will in due time pass away with the instinct that is its support, leaving only the love of God and the calm bliss belonging to it, which instinct may be likened to a night-watchman, who, when he sees the dawn, awakens the day-watchman and then disappears. He says: "As the love of God grows in the soul the human love cools and is forgotten". The transition he speaks of as a severe discipline. The devotee is apt to become discouraged and fear he is not serving God. John of the Cross, as Madam Guyon does too, speaks of a season of purgative aridity or "spiritual dryness", and says, "the cause of this dryness is that God is transferring to the spirit the goods and energies of the senses". Said a lady who had just visited a convent: "You needn't tell me those nuns, so sleek and plump, placid and contented, are old maids". Of course the remark was purely absurd, as probably it was thoughtless. She might have been told that those pleasant-faced inmates enjoyed a compensation in their single-blessedness that spinsters of the outer world know nothing of. Probably the flagellated ladies mentioned in Von Ebing's book had, long before they shouted in their ecstasy, passed into the state where all love is God-love, and love of man but rudimental. Yet both are physical and have the same physical support, and are not always separate in their activities, if John of the Cross is good authority. He says, in treating of the strange impure experiences that result from their mingling with or overlapping one another: " They proceed occasionally — though but rarely and in persons of delicate constitution — from sensible sweetness in spiritual things. For when sense and spirit are both united together, the whole nature of man is moved in that delectation, according to its measure and character. For then the spirit, that is the higher part of our nature, is moved to delight itself in God; and sensuality, which is the lower part, is moved towards sensible gratification, because it knows and admits of none other".

Further proof of the close kindred of the two loves is found in the fact that both are subject to the same kind of perversion, or, as distinguished alienists insist, insanity. Of late years Doctor Moll of Berlin, Doctor Von Kraft Ebing of Vienna and others by their researches and writings have made known to the world the character of certain anomalous manifestations of the sexual instinct concerning which, though of too common occurrence, little or nothing was before known, and which, when noticed at all, were treated as crimes. One of these to which has been given the name of masochism is described by Von Kraft Ebing as "that particular perversion of the psychic vita sexualis which consists in the fact that the individual is, in his feelings and in his sexual thoughts, possessed by the idea of being subjected absolutely and unconditionally to a person of the other sex, to be treated by that person in a haughty manner, even to the point of inflicting humiliation and torture. The idea is accompanied by voluptuous sensations; he who is smitten with it loves to imagine scenes of the above sort and often tries to realize them, and, by such perversion of his sexual tendency becomes frequently more or less insensible to the normal charms of the other sex, incapable of a normal vita sexualis, psychically impotent. This psychic impotence, however, is nowise based on the horror sexualis alterius j it is founded on the fact that the satisfaction of the perverse tendency can, as in normal cases, come from the woman, but not from connection with her".

One masochist who wrote out full details of his own case and those of others, adds the following: " Men attainted with this perversion submit themselves to the most refined tortures. With women trained to it the same comedy is gone through with at each visit; the man humbly prostrates himself ; then there are kicks, imperious commands, insults and threats that have been learned by heart; then whipping, blows on divers parts of the body and all kinds of tortures, pricking with pins till blood comes, etc". " At two different times prostitutes have shown me chains of iron with handcuffs that their clients had had made to be used on themselves, also dried peas for them to kneel on, cushions bristling with needles upon which they must sit when ordered to do so, and many other things of like sort".

Another wrote down for the benefit of a fellow masochist a set of instructions in twenty paragraphs, telling how he should get himself treated as a slave and tortured. Another used to go once a week to a certain kind of house and hire three of the heaviest of the women to trample on him for hours, which was all he required of them. And as to dirtiness it is said that cases are not rare of masochists who procured themselves to be befouled in all imaginable ways, even to the extent of matching in that respect "the Christian ecstatic Antoinette Bouvignon of La Porte, who mixed excrement with her food in order to mortify herself, and Marie Alacoque, since beatified, who for her mortification licked the dejections of sick persons and sucked their great toes covered with sores".

As cruelty to one's self naturally runs into cruelty to others, it is not surprising that masochism is often allied to another congenital anomaly or perversion of the sexual nature, called sadism, and which calls for every degree of cruelty from wringing the neck of a chicken to murdering a mistress, cutting her up, drinking her blood and eating her flesh, a la mode Jack the Ripper of Whitechapel. One beginning as a sadist will be apt to develop as a masochist, and vice versa. "Sadism", remarks Von Kraft Ebing, "is the very opposite of masochism. While the one wants to endure pain, and feel himself subjugated, the other seeks to produce suffering and violence. The parallelism is complete. All the acts and all the scenes which are performed by the sadist in an active way constitute the object of the desires of the masochist in his passive role. In the two perversions these acts progress gradually from symbolic presentations to the worst tortures. Even assassination from a voluptuous impulse, the acme of sadism, finds its passive counterpart at least in imaginings. Both perversions can, circumstances favoring, exist side by side with a normal vita sexualis; in both the acts by which they manifest themselves serve to render possible what was before impossible, or else serve as substitutes for it. The analogy concerns not only the external symptoms, but extends to the inner essence of the two perversions; which must equally be considered as psychopathic and congenital in certain individuals whose psychic states are abnormal, and who are above all afflicted with hyperesthesia sexualis".

And now taking sadism and masochism thus rolled into one, and comparing the one perversion of the lower or man love which they represent with the perversion so often manifesting itself in ascetics of the higher or God love, we see that there are common to both of them the three elements of cruelty, humiliation and dirt as producers of certain sensations, which flow directly from them and without calling into use the physical apparatus already rendered useless by the practice of austerities, or resulting from what is by our author termed psychic impotence ; and seeing that cruelty, humiliation and dirt is all there is in either form of perverted love, the resemblance amounts to identity. This conclusion exonerates the religious principle from being considered the cause of the maniacal doings of ascetics of any faith. But it does not exonerate from blame a church who exhibits as her best work such specimens as sainted Simeon Stylites, Mary of Egypt, John of the Cross and Blessed Marie Alacoque, wretches who by reason of some anomalous congenital perversion of their psychic natures were unable to get by harmless or decent modes of contemplation the blissful sensations they craved anymore than the sadists and masochists, afflicted by a like perversion, can obtain in a natural way those they crave, and by a like insane impulsion with theirs are driven to the very same vile practices.

The masochist, psychically impuissant, the worn-out debauchee, physically so, and the ascetic, unable otherwise to attain to the saintly ecstasy known as the love of God, all flagellate themselves on the same part; which certainly seems to prove that the higher love depends on the same physical apparatus as the lower, and is not an independent emotion of the soul.

The analogy existing between masochism and sadism, on the one hand, and cruel religious penance on the other, which consists in this, that all of them aim at bringing pleasure out of pain, has not escaped Doctor Von Kraft Ebing. But certainly the resemblance which another sexual perversion described by him, and named fetichism, bears to relic worship is strong enough to justify a serious belief that the latter grew out of the former. In one subject to fetichism, "the sexual interest is concentrated exclusively on a determinate part of the body of a woman or on certain parts of feminine apparel". Impelled by a delirious instinct, the fetichist ravishes, not the woman herself, but a lock of her hair, a shoe or a handkerchief, and in caressing his plunder obtains all the satisfaction another could have had from possessing her person.

To the attraction of physical pleasure, not doubtful or distant, but certain and immediate, and waited on by an instinctual impulse that will not be refused, every man owes his being. And if Nature, having brought his race thus far along the path of evolution, intends to allure it further, it will be by analogous means, we may be sure. But it is her habit to improve her methods as she goes; and what is the most obvious improvement on the old and lower love unless it be the new and the higher of which we have got glimpses while searching out the secrets of yoga? If this be so, then according to all analogy and precedent the later love must be a projection of

223

the earlier on the same lines with it, and, moreover, the mechanism that has heretofore served the one, must so far as applicable, do duty for the other.

Has Nature, creative Nature, any further work to do on man?

Union

Teachers of the different schools of yoga agree well enough concerning observable results, but when they go beyond them and undertake to know what happens to the yogi after he attains, into what state of being he passes, they get beyond their depth and float in the sea called speculative philosophy, wherein each swims his own way. All tell of an union, but concerning what is united to what, and in what manner, they differ widely. The Hindus make the union to consist in an eternal identity with Brahman, and attainment to consist in thoroughly knowing it. The Egyptians made of it nothing more than a temporary assimilation with some personal god, for magical purposes. The Christians talk of an union with God, which is yet no union at all, but merely a presence. He being of a nature too high to unite with man's. Ancient Akkadian magic united the practicer of it to a being variously apprehended as a part of liis own soul, his type or essence, or his guardian spirit or divinity. Taoism, whose god was a principle, had an at-one-ment with it attainable by the man, "whose physical frame is perfect and whose vitality is in its original purity" — something quite different from the final return of him to the source whence he came. Taoism seems to have looked in the very opposite direction from absorption, as will appear further on, under the heading of Perfection.

Neoplatonism, too, had its own peculiar union, which was brief, occasional and made no final disposition of the soul. The soul, always in a certain sense in God, got no nearer to him in life or death than when from time to time it attained to what John of the Cross calls "touches of union",

described by him as being so delightful and by Plotinus so delightfully described. Always homesick for its native sky, and having received from pitying Jupiter the gift of mortality, it habitually returned there to dwell between its re-incarnations.

All beliefs that have arisen out of yoga experience, whether justly or erroneously, were the best, the wisest, men of the times could formulate, and have value as indications of what those experiences really were. Thus the diverse beliefs concerning the kind of union that rewards the attaining yogi's pains, while by their diversity they make it impossible for more than one of them to be true, and cast great doubt on that, yet by their agreement, so far as they do agree, tend to prove that among those experiences are physical sensations or mental impressions as of something coming into closer relations than it had before with another something. Such might be the rapprochement of the normal centre of consciousness and the nerve-centres, or of the normal volition and the socalled involuntary muscles, or of whatever stands for soul with the body it pertains to, whether that be a resultant of material forces, as the materialists claim, or a sky-born entity that descends into generation more or less deep according as it sees the body to need its presence, as a Neoplatonist would have said.

In what has just been stated of six theories relating to union, it is seen that only one of them, Vedantin Hinduism, attempts to unfold the final destiny of the soul, which it does by leading it back to whence it came and leaving it there for a Hindu eternity, while another, old Taoism, as if it held earth-life to be all, or at least as ignoring every other, points towards an infinite enlargement of that as man's destiny, to attain to which however, it is forward, not backward, he is to go, and the material earth that he is to tread. Thus these two great systems teach doctrines as opposite to each other as they very well can, and which tend mutually to discredit each other, since both rest on like authority, namely, mystical experience, intuition, revelation. But so far as primitive yoga literature discloses, old Hinduism was as careless of the soul's destiny apart from that of the body as old Taoism was, and looked as exclusively towards the earth as the home of the united two. The modern commentator on Swatmaram's book says of Hatha Yoga : " It even bestows the gift of putting off death indefinitely" ; in which he is in agreement with vulgar belief in India at the present time. Besides the statement before quoted concerning the thirty-five gods and yogis, Swatmaram's book contains the following promises of longevity at least as the reward of yoga practice: "And the yogi lives long "; " becomes a lad of sixteen, ever free from old age"; "even poison itself proves to him but nectar"; "the yogi becomes young, though old "; "a yogi in Samadhi is invulnerable to all weapons".

But the following certainly mean more than longevity: " The Yogi cheats death "; "These are the ten Mudras that destroy old age and death"; "This Maha Mudra destroys death "; "This frees one from the great noose of King Yama " (death); "These three Bandhas that ward off death and old age" ; " To him who knows the Khechari Mudra there is no disease or death, and Time has no power over him"; "(This act) enables him to ward off weapons of every sort, confers on him immortality"; " He who practices this for three hours daily conquers death", "even though he is in the mouth of death, he need not fear it"; "He conquers Time (death) playfully"; "Salutations to you, Amaras (immortals) by whom Time, into whose mouth the universe falls, has been conquered"; "Death is not experienced by the practicer of this Mudra"; "The man perfect in Rajah Yoga deceives death"; "A Yogi in Samadhi is not destroyed by death"; "is invulnerable to all weapons"; "Brahman and Gods devoting themselves to the practice of Pranyama were freed from the fear of death". One verse undertakes to explain how it is that man is subject to death and another to explain why his body becomes old, by the fact that " every particle of nectar (the Satravi) that flows from the Ambrosial Moon is swallowed up by the Sun", an explanation which the commentator says is purposely absurd; but the offering of which indicates that the sages claimed to have knowledge of the causes of old age and death and also of processes by which their action could be annulled.

These many allusions to immortality found in a hundred-page volume are not contradicted by anything else it contains save one or two phrases in which may imply deliverance from re-incarnation, of which I have before said that they are so inconsistent with the whole tenor of the book that they probably are interpolations. The immortality intended in the passages quoted is to be acquired by the yogi's own efforts, something not predicable of incorporeal immortality, since all conceptions of that include a soul capable, to be sure, of being punished or rewarded after its body's death, but itself incapable of dying; a soul whose persistence does not depend on its possessor's efforts, but is his in spite of anything he can do or omit. So that the immortality in question can be no other than corporeal. Nor can it be construed to signify an indefinitely prolonged life, for the words used will bear no such limitation.

New Birth

This term occurs so often in the literature of magic that there must be something in the experiences of magicians to suggest it. Yet no writer reveals just what that something is, nor just how the term applies to it. The same may be said of the often-occurring word regeneration, which may be intended as synonymous with re-birth, though it comes nearer to re-begetting. Both are often repeated in Christian writings. Methodistical Protestants attach the same meaning to them that they do to "finding Jesus", "getting religion" or "having a change of heart", terms as badly in want of definition as themselves. As commonly used, they signify to Christians an improvement in the moral disposition such as Protestants of that sort are said to undergo between conversion and backsliding; but perhaps love experiences of some kind may be at the bottom. In any case it behooves the student of magic to follow the clew the words new birth and regeneration tender.

Perfection

To John of the Cross this word signified union with God, and such must be taken to be the Church's construction of the perfection to which Jesus attained through suffering and which he promised his disciples they should also reach. The gnostics and Kabbalists held that perfection was arrived at by means of successive re-incarnations. The Greeks named their mysteries "Tellai", which means perfection. The alchemists of Christian times taught " that man was perfectible and in the scheme of nature destined to and bound for perfection", and that so was everything else in nature, whose imperfect work their art occupied itself with amending. Old Taoism makes perfection, the perfection of the man of the earth and for purposes of earth-life, the object and aim of magical practice — quite a different one, as said before, from that of Vedantism, which is the getting away from that life by getting to God. The one contemplates the completion of an unfinished piece of creative work; the other the abandoning it. The one points forward along an unending way to infinite excellence; the other points backward towards the starting point of a sad, unprofitable journey.

To the Taoist the words saint, sage and perfect man meant one and the same thing, and it was Taoism's greatest saint and sage and most perfect man who said : " Tao conducts to perfection". That this perfection was of the earthly body and being is declared plainly enough by his greatest disciple Chuang-Tzü in the following passages: "See nothing, hear nothing, let your soul be wrapped in quiet; and your body will begin to take the proper form. Let there be absolute repose and absolute purity, do not weary your body nor disturb your vitality — and you will live forever. For if the eye sees nothing and the ear hears nothing and the mind thinks nothing, the soul will preserve the body and the body will live forever".

"Cherish and preserve your own self".

"I preserve the original one while resting in harmony with eternals. It is because I have thus cared for myself during twelve hundred years that my body has not decayed".

" By renouncing the world one gets rid of the cares of the world. The result is a natural level, which is equivalent to a re-birth. And he who is re-born is near".

"But why renounce the affairs of men and become indifferent to life ? In the first case his physical body suffers no wear and tear; in the second the vitality is left unimpaired. And he whose physical frame is perfect and whose vitality is in its original purity, he is at one with Heaven".

"But if body and vitality are both perfect, this state is called fit for translation".

"And if I can refrain from injuring my animal economy and from taxing my powers of sight and hearing, sitting like a corpse while my dragon-power is manifested around — in profound silence while my thunder voice resounds, the powers of heaven responding to every phase of my will, as under the gentle influence of inaction all things are brought to maturity and thrive — what leisure have I then to set about governing the world?"

Concerning other magical powers of the perfected man Chuang-Tzü says:

" His knowledge extends to the supernatural.'

" If men are without Tao, by a mere look he calls them to a sense of error". And finally and inclusively we have this sweeping clause: "Once attain to Tao, and there is nothing which you cannot accomplish"

That the Taoists believed in a past Golden Age, when men were morally perfect, appears from the following: "In the Golden Age rulers were mere beacons. The people were free as wild deer. They were upright without being conscious of duty to their neighbor. They loved one another without being conscious of charity. They were true without being conscious of loyalty. They were honest without being conscious of good faith. They acted freely in all things without recognizing obligation to any one. Thus their deeds left no trace and their affairs were not handed down to posterity".

From their belief in a past Golden Age the Taoists may well enough have derived the expectation of one in the future, and also the idea of man's perfectibility. That they, like the old Hindu sages, had notions of the evolution of man from the lower orders of creation, much like those now so largely occupying the minds of our scientific men, and from thence inferred an indefinite continuance of his progress in the direction of perfection, and that consciously, is shown by the following saying of Chuang-Tzü : "To have attained to the human form must be always a source of joy. And then to'undergo countless transitions with only the infinite to look forward to — what incomparable bliss is that ! " Words like these could hardly apply to a series of evolutionary changes, each one cut off from the others by death and oblivion, as has been the case in the past.

CHAPTER XXVIII - EARTHLY IMMORTALITY

The immortality which, according to the ancient Taoist and Hindu sages, was attainable through yoga practice was not entered upon through the gates of death nor enjoyed in the skies, neither in the land of the fathers nor in the land of the gods, nor in the bosom of Brahman. The possessor of it was, according to the Taoists, one who had undergone transformation, not dissolution, "fit for translation" from here, but still here ; according to the Hindus, "moving about the world". It was accompanied by an equipment of magical qualities, the Siddhis, adapted to and necessary to it, and not adapted to any other conceivable mode of existence than in a physical body and on a material earth. For mortal man they have hitherto at least proved of small use for good. Although beyond measure wonderful, they are as yet quantitatively scant. We do not learn that the experiment of the good Chinese emperor in governing by magic resulted in the permanent abolition of rulers and laws, though one is tempted to wish it had. The success of Elijah in calling down flame from Heaven to kindle his altar fagots did not dispense with any of the other tiresome methods of starting fires that taxed the sweat of men before tinder, flint and steel were brought into use by the practical kind of magic called invention. Spectres of gods and men have been exhibited by theurgists and necromancers, but it is not probable that any theatrical company was ever made up of spectral illusions. Real flowers often fall from the ceiling upon the seance-table, but never in quantity adequate to the requirements of a fashionable funeral. Just before a memorable panic in Wall Street, a certain speculator was by an invisible hand pushed in the direction of his broker's office, while a voice in his ear said : " Go and close up your margins", which, neglecting to do, he was ruined on " Black Friday", yet his experience has failed to furnish any sure way of knowing in advance how the market will turn, and with him all the thousands of other "operators for a rise" on that same day went unadmonished to pecuniary perdition. Abaris, the Celtic priest of Apollo, when on a visit to Pythagoras, crossed a river astride an arrow, and Elijah, by threshing with his mantle the waters of Jordan, caused them to part and let him pass over dry-shod, yet no ferry has yet been worked on the principle of levitation, nor any stream been made permanently fordable by Elijah's method. Magical healers have always abounded, yet none the less so have medicinal ones. Fortune-tellers tell fortunes truly, yet still the future is dark. And without ignoring the benefits that have undoubtedly been derived from magic, yet, considering the disturbance it has caused in the world as it is, one may easily see that the world as it is would have been better without it — which is the commonest and also the best argument that is urged against magical studies. And a perception of the inadaptability of magic to our actual life is probably at the bottom of the rather stolid disregard of it in modern times. Hindu philosophy, which includes that of Buddhism and therefore covers nearly all of Asia, rejects the Siddhis as worthless for the saint and dangerous if possessed by the sinner, howbeit there, as elsewhere and always, religion puts a portion of them to its own use, and diverts Prana, the life-breath, to blow upon the mill-wheels that grind the grist of the priests.

Of European mankind the Catholic part are allowed to do nothing in magic except under Church surveillance, that follows into his locked cell the ascetic who retires there, in the words of Plotinus, " to receive God and to be alone with the Alone " — and grimly presides over his meditations. All of magic, beyond the small portion appropriated and controlled by the Church, is jumped up and down upon by both it and the State. The Protestant part, having been told by Luther that the day of magic was past, quite ignores it, except that occasionally it is allowed to play the part of the "inner witness", a kind of professional witness, and a willing one, that most always testifies in favor of the party calling it. And so it is that there is small use or place for magic in the world as it is.

Difficulties in the Way

Even if Nature should effect in the organism the proper change (possibly a very slight one) needed to secure to the individual man what may be termed physiological immortality, good against death by old age, yet disease would remain ; if he were rendered pathologically immortal by the extinction of disease, there would still he hard rocks for him to fall on, or to fall on him, water to drown and fire to consume him, cold to freeze and famine to starve, ferocious beasts to eat, machinery to crush, gases to suffocate, and elemental violence of every kind to overwhelm and sweep him into the gaping hopper of death. After long and hard battling with these, and thereby proving himself fit to live, warrantable to last with good usage some seventy years or so, man remains at present date a very perishable article, vulnerable still to his old enemies. Two sages, at least, both of them believers in terrestrial immortality, have shown in their writings that they foresaw these difficulties in the way of it, by suggesting methods for overcoming them. Says Chuang-Tzu: " The perfect man can walk through solid bodies without obstruction. He can pass through fire without being burnt. He can scale the greatest heights without fear".

" He could ride upon the wind and travel whithersoever he wished, staying away as long as fifteen days".

"The perfect man is a spiritual being. Were the ocean half scorched up he would not feel hot. Were the milky way frozen over he would not feel cold. Were the mountains riven with thunder and the great deep upheaved by storm he would not tremble. In such case he would mount upon the clouds of heaven, and, driving the sun and moon before him, would pass beyond the limits of this external world to where death and life themselves have no more victory over man".

It was a long while after Chuang-Tzü that Jacob Boehme wrote the following: "Before his fall, man could rule over the sun and the stars. Everything was in his power. Fire, air, water and earth could not tame him; no fire burned him, no water drowned, no air suffocated him; all that lived stood in awe of him".

" No heat, no cold, no sickness nor accident, nor any fear could touch or terrify him. His body could pass through earth and rocks without breaking anything in them, for a man who could be overpowered by the terrestrial nature would not be eternal".

What has last been quoted from Chuang-Tzü complements what was quoted from him under the head of Perfection, which by itself and on a first reading may seem to make immortality depend on continual care of the body and to ignore the necessity of the magical qualities as its support and protection, the two quotations taken together, however, amounting to a distinct declaration of a doctrine of physiological and pathological immortality protected and supported by Siddhis conferring invulnerability, etc. Indeed, the first quotation may be said to imply the need of these adjuncts, as, for instance, where the words, "it is because I have thus cared for myself during twelve hundred years that my body has not decayed", are followed by "the result is a natural level, which is equivalent to a re-birth. And he who is re-born is near"; and soon afterward by these : "But if body and vitality both are perfect this state is called fit for translation". Mere physiological and pathological longevity, dependent on persistent care of the body, cannot be the state here referred to, and we must presume a radical and permanent transformation rendering death from any cause impossible to be intended.

The idea of immortality thus held up as a reward of diligent yoga practice, whether capable of being realized or not, need not hide its head in presence of any other yet devised by human ingenuity; it looks in the only direction our minds are able to turn, points to the only way our feet are fitted to travel and promises the only kind of life we know how to live. Let us, therefore, not disdain to go further in the examination of the grounds of it, and to that end, of the adaptability to a state of being which is nothing else than immortality in the flesh and on the earth, of the Siddhis that attend its attainment (including in that term all magical powers possible to man, or believed by the sages to be so). A reference to the statements of the nature these, as given by Lao-Tsee and Chuang-Tzü and the Hatha and Vedanta schools, will show that both the Hindu and Taoist authorities, to say nothing of others, substantially concur in making of them a complete suit of armor to defend the immortal against the following evils expected to beset him even after becoming exempt from death by old age:

1. All other effects of age. 2. Disease. 3. Poison. 4. Impact of solid bodies, thus of all kinds of physical violence. 5. Fire. 6. Water. 7. Suffocating gases and vapors. 8. Imprisonment and other personal restraint. 9. Hunger, thirst and all forms of poverty. 10. Evil magic. The qualities requisite to meet these dangers may be summarized as follows:

1. Immunity from wear and tear: Magical writings abound in accounts of prolonged youth and even actual rejuvenescence, from Moses, whose "eye was not dimmed, nor his natural force abated", when at the age of an hundred and twenty he disappeared, to Postel's nun, who when nearing sixty looked fifteen.

2. Unlimited receptivity to the ever-superabundant flow of vital force, ready and pressing to enter, must needs exclude all forms of disease.

3. Immunity from venomous reptiles: Saint Paul was not the only magician that a snake-bite could not kill; thousands of such now live.

4. The permeability of matter: That matter can pass through matter unhurting and unhurt is now being proved in many a circle of modern Spiritualists, especially in America. Jesus of Nazareth is said to have gone in and out through closed doors, in his earthly body of solid flesh, and Apollonius of Tyania and Saint Peter escaped, the one from arrest and the other from prison, in the same way. This permeability of matter is, however, but slowly getting believed in even by the experimenters themselves, and this notwithstanding modern science has come to its aid by proving that, after all, the final atoms into which matter can be resolved are only vortices of ether whirling at a distance each from the others, and that ether is not material — thus that the hardest rock is but a mist of atomized motion.

5. Incombustibility: Many who are willing to admit that in this generation the medium Home more than once handled live coals of fire, and that in some eastern countries devotees, prepared for the purpose by a course of fasting and prayer, walk barefoot over beds of them, would shrink from accepting as literally true the story of Shadrach, Meshac and Abednego going through a superheated furnace, yet in all the cases the principle involved is the same. In normal conditions, to expose hands or feet to the action of fire without getting them burnt is impossible; and that is the worst can be said of walking through a furnace, however fiery.

6. Levitation: One able to rise and float in the air, after the manner of Elijah, Simon Magus and the medium Home, need not drown in water. And levitation of men and furniture is nowadays both common and cheap.

7. Ability to live without breathing : Suffocation should be impossible to a yogi who has learned to do without breathing through performing the Khechari Mudra.

8. Absolute freedom of locomotion: No prison or fetters could restrain a magician able to pass through matter like those who have been named.

9. Abundant wealth: Poverty could certainly have no place in a world peopled by magicians able, like Jesus and Elijah, to multiply food at discretion, or like many an Indian faquir, to raise a tree from the seed in a few minutes' time.

10. Inaccessibility to malignant spells: Evil magicians vainly aim their enchantments against an attained yogi; as Plotinus puts it: "A self-centred man cannot be bewitched". It may be suggested that an easier way than the above to render a man indestructible would be to let him die, and in his spirit body, a duplicate of the physical one, go and dwell forever in a spirit world, a duplicate of this physical earth. But would he not be assailed there by exact duplicates of every destructive agency that menaced him here, as well adapted to work on the spirit body as they on the natural one ?

Again it may be suggested, all the physiologically immortal man would need to render him actually deathproof would be a knowledge of the future, the remote and the hidden, such as would forewarn him of approaching danger and teach him how to avoid it. But this would make his life dependent on his own vigilance andvolition; and Nature's habit is not to trust the preservation of her work to anything so precarious as these if she can do better, as she does in placing the vegetative movements of the organism, the breathing, circulation, etc., under the control of the involuntary muscles. In fact the difficulty in question applies to some of the siddhis themselves, which would be of no use without the action of the will, as for instance the power of levitation and that of doing without breath, the mere possession of which, without the will to exert them at the proper time would still leave the individual exposed to death by drowning or suffocation by noxious air, or want of air. But to meet these difficulties all needed would be such a transformation as would place all movement requisite to preserve life under the control of the involuntary and unconscious part of man, just as the vegetative movements now are — although Hindu philosophers say that once it was not so, and claim it to be proved by the fact that some yogis have regained the original voluntary control over certain organs, and can even arrest the beating of the heart at will. Certainly if, as many wise men have believed, man made himself, he must have begun by functioning each organ voluntarily and consciously, and continued to do so until by long practice the proper movement became habitual, automatic, and went on independently of his will or thought. To many, perhaps to most persons, this would be inconceivable ; but to one who will scan the progress of man's creation upward from the worm that had the honor to be his ancestor, whatever may be his opinion concerning the kind of agency operating it, whether supernatural or mechanical, it ought not to be so, nor should such an one distrust the cunning of the hand that did the work, or doubt its ability to carry it on. And it may even be possible to some speculative minds to conjecture that the future progress of the race may be through a series of transitions from voluntary activities to involuntary ones, the voluntary being first set up by the conscious brain and when perfected by that, remitted to the control of the unconscious one, or of the little brains which the nerve-centres are, while the conscious man passes on to the work of self-perfection next in order. One consequence of such a state of things might be that men would remit to the control of the unconscious the more distasteful of the activities of life — perhaps all of them, and like Krishna, god, yogi and warrior, who declared that while he was cutting and thrusting in the hot of the battle his consciousness of his own exploits was only that of a witness, and not of a doer.

If at a time before the first human being appeared, and while as yet the anthropoid ape was at the head of the column and lord of creation, that animal had considered the possibility of his place being taken by so poor a sort of ape as man, of a creature so soft being able to live in a world so hard as this, when even he, with his tough and shaggy hide, long arms, strong claws and great jaws, had to struggle to hold his own, he would, probably, have seen serious difficulties in the way of such possibility, and dismissed the subject from consideration as contemptuously as he would have regarded the idea of there being needed at the head of the column any better lord of creation than himself. And it would not be strange if members of the race that has displaced the ape should see many more difficulties than those which have been suggested in the way of any of themselves dwelling in deathless persistence on this earth that has so long been much more their burial-place than dwelling-place. But more than a difficulty is involved in the questions at once arising: Whereabouts in the world do yogis who have become immortal, keep themselves ? Why do they shun intercourse with us poor mortals, their descendants, so greatly needing the aid and guidance of their superior power and intelligence ? Or is their philosophical equanimity so perfect that human concerns no longer interest them, and they still remain in that state of stupidity in which, as John of the Cross says, the Christian contemplative has miraculous aid from his God in attending to his temporal affairs, but for which purpose the Hindus say any careful man will do ? Or are they, on the other hand, wise enough to know the secrets of nature and that all is going on as well as it can, and also know themselves too ignorant to judge the scheme of the universe, or shake the jar wherein human destiny is solving itself ? To keep out of the way do they magically render themselves invisible to mortal sight, or take themselves out of reach of any mortal sense, by rising in the air as Elijah did, or like Moses burying themselves — performing the Khechari Mudra, and with tongues uprolled hybernating in inaccessible caves ?

But, notwithstanding the peculiar adaptation of the Siddhis in their possible unlimited development to rendering possible terrestrial immortality, and of those just mentioned to keeping mortals separate from immortals during a supposable transitional period in which both should inhabit the same earth, one of them, invisibility, being apparently of no use for any other purpose, the only safe conclusion is a denial that any such immortals exist.

But such a conclusion must still leave the Siddhis as well proved as before — and as unexplained. Had our race ever been endowed with immortality they would have been essential supports to it; if it is destined ever to be so endowed, they are a needed preparation for it; if either is to come before the other, it is, of course, the preparation, and not the thing prepared for. It makes for nothing against the reality of the Siddhis that the state of being they are adapted to has not yet arrived, though it makes for much in favor of the future realization of it that they have come, or are coming, in quantity however scant as yet, while their adaptation to it makes them the logical harbingers of it. Thus the reasons hereinbefore supposed to have caused in the Taoist and Hindu sages' minds the belief that some of their number had already achieved immortality of the sort in question, namely, the adaptation to it of magically obtained immunity from bodily wear and tear, disease, poison, violence, accidental burning, freezing, drowning, suffocation, crushing byrocks, poverty and evil magic, though failing to justify the belief in question, stand nevertheless good for the supposition that the possession of, or ability to acquire such immunity, evinces Nature's intent at some epoch, in the future to bring about the state of things for which it will come in play. The way Nature faces she will surely go. Her intention can be inferred from her acts. Do her acts allow us to expect her next step to be in the direction of making this earth man's permanent home ? A population of reproductive immortals no globe could long contain. A world without love no one would wish to inhabit for any life term — long or short. The Taoist and Hindu yogis lately quoted do not seem to have considered these two little difficulties. Swedenborg did, and avoided them by allowing his immortals to beget as many "goods and truths " as they should desire to beget, instead of children. But if certain strenuously asserted facts are true, a better plan has been devised by Nature, which is this: Along with the Siddhis, and as results of the same course of practice which produces them, there comes sterility to man and barrenness to woman, from whom both her curse and lesser curse take themselves away forever. See again what has been quoted from Saint John of the Cross concerning the dying out of the natural, and the arising in its place of the spiritual love; also what has been quoted concerning the "secret or mysterious love " of the Sufis, concerning the "amatory mania" mentioned with so much respect by Plato, and about Krishna, whose twelve thousand human misery no longer touches their hearts ? Or do wives, for whom he multiplied himself into twelve thousand husbands, lauded his complaisance as all the more wonderful for the reason that being a god he needed no human mate, having all joy within himself, and other passages having a direct or indirect bearing on the important bodily transformation in question.

CHAPTER XXIX - YOGA AS A PROCESS OF EVOLUTION

In the mind of him who observes the course of man's evolution in the past, and judges Nature's intention by her acts, three presumptions will arise,

1. That because this material globe has hitherto been the scene of operations, it will continue to be so henceforth. 2. That because the beginning was indefinitely long ago, the end will be indefinitely long hence. 3. That because the transformations have until now been from the less perfect to the more perfect, with a general tendency, at least, toward the avoidance of evil and attainment of good, man's destiny is to continually become more perfect and more happy, though probably never absolutely so. These constitute, as it seems to me, a presumption in favor of a happy immortality being in store for man upon the earth where he was born and has always dwelt, so strong as to put on the defensive every theory to the contrary. Of the slime of that earth the egg of his beginning was formed, in its mud as a worm he crawled, in its waters as a fish he swam, in its forests and on its mountains as a mammal he foraged for fruits and nuts, or killed and ate or was killed or eaten. And now, after having during a course of time infinitely long attained to a state wherein he can turn and lay his creative hand on it, make its surface productive and its aspect beautiful, open roadways and water-ways to bring all its parts into neighborhood, control its floods and pierce its rocks; why should he not, as mortal or immortal and through all future changes continue where he is?

During incalculable time animal life has, by successive growths, produced man, each growth consisting of a new species produced from the one next preceding it. Some of these species have in course of time disappeared, while some remain; but hitherto the existence of none of them has required the extinction of any other, and without serious hindrance to man a vast population of fishes, reptiles, birds and beasts, some lineal and others collaterally related to him, occupy the same globe with him; but how will it be in the future ? Judging by analogy, man should produce, when progress resumes its march, a race superior to him, and this another superior to it, and so on, growth after growth, reaching as indefinitely far into time to come as the procession at his back reaches into time gone, and developing stage by stage into something as superior to him as the worm is inferior. And whether each race is, as some suppose, doomed after reaching its prime to degenerate, or is destined to continually perfect itself, the existence of any one of them comtemporaneously with any other would seem to be impossible, even were the contemporaries the present man and his immediate successor; much more so the existence of an indefinitely numerous congress of such unequally developed races.

Evidently, if evolution is to go any further, there must be a change of method.

Natural selection which, according to Wallace, has hitherto done all, but according to Darwin only part, of the work on man — a process of exhaustive reproduction and wasteful slaughter — is a principle that must always operate while the population of the globe consists of procreating mortals; yet it is not itself exempt from the law of evolution. As the agency for carrying the race further on the way to perfection, it may have to yield place to the slower, more interior method of transformation, which yoga is. In fact, the development of man from the ape, the links needed to prove which to have been done by natural selection are still missing, though searched for from cellar to garret, may have been the work of yoga. Just how nature will manage it all is her own secret, but a guess may be ventured that it will be by the simple process of transforming the race from a mortal into an immortal state of being, as the sages of old insisted had in numerous cases already been done, but which, for reasons before stated, it is safer to look for as yet to be done, if to be done ever. Such a process would comport with nature's well-known habits of economizing force, going to her ends by the shortest way, moving on lines of least resistance, taking advantage of favoring winds, currents and other accidents, using old material so far as applicable, and preferring to graft the buds of differentiation on stocks already existing to uprooting and planting anew, and is, in fact, her habit in the evolution of the foetus. Thus would death be cast into the same pit where hell is already tumbling, death fulfilling scripture by going in last.

A world of such immortals, enjoying perpetual youth and beauty and all the magical qualities and powers of which the Siddhis are but the rudiments, where, in the absence of old age, infancy and disease, there would be no poverty or crime, laws or rules, nor aught to hinder freedom, where, if labor should be found inconvenient, all the movements of it could be transferred to the jurisdiction of the unconscious mind, as has been done with the vegetative movements of the body, and in the same automatic, habitual infallible way that these are per formed all wants supplied; or where, instead of this, all ills of life possible to an immortal could be nullified by his simply lapsing into that state of apathetic equanimity wherein even the spectacle of the sacking of a city would in no wise annoy him — such a world would, at first thought, seem to human reason above criticism. Yet there is room for cavil after all; would it not be a tiresome world?

Death, in the sense of final annihilation, if such can be, cannot be called an evil, for, as the stoic said: "Where I am death is not, and where death is I am not". But all men can foresee that soon or late the tedium of the most paradisical existence must convert itself into torment. Now this last difficulty was plainly foreseen and provided for in both the old Taoist and Hindu systems. The Hindu immortal could die at will, and go to Brahman ; and the mere knowledge of this, it is conceivable, might make it agreeable to continue in life, just as one in a box with a lid loosely laid on might comfortably and quietly remain there for hours, and even fall asleep, but should others attempt to screw down the lid, would yell in agony and struggle with all his might to get out. But better than the power to die at will was the promise held out to the Taoist saint, of undying change, each transition being from good to better, for such is the meaning of the notable words of Chuang-Tsü, already quoted, but worth many times quoting: "To have attained to the human form must always be a source of joy. And then to undergo countless transitions, with only the infinite to look forward to — what incomparable bliss is that! "

Here is no revelation, no outgiving of mystical intuition — neither Lao-Tsee nor his disciple had to do with such — but simply the statement of an inference of the human reason, drawn from the analogies of nature, and which presupposes a knowledge of the evolution of man in a like way obtained.

That man, considered as a physical organism, after undergoing an indefinite number of transitions bringing him up to what he now is, should be destined to undergo an indefinite number more, carrying him still farther on the way to perfection, should seem to us not absurd, but most reasonable rather, even though we cannot so much as dream what they are to be or whither lead, while all concern we may feel about nature's ability to effect them in some way or other of her own ought to be quieted by a glance backward at what she has already achieved. No one can give a reason why the chain of causation should stop at man that would not also be a reason for its stopping at the ape, to whose comprehension his destiny to evolve into man could have got no access, any more than man's destiny to become something as superior to what he now is, as he is now superior to the ape, to become immortal in the flesh, could be grasped by his.

However all this may be, do not these theories of old China and India show better grounds for themselves than any others that have got into vogue, relating to man's destiny? In all others, terrestrial immortality not being supposed, there is necessarily introduced the supposition of a soul capable of existence separate from a body, and this is what Kant demonstrated could not be demonstrated, owing to the forms of knowledge of the human intellect. But supposing it proved, in any of the modes hitherto relied on, there would still remain to be answered the question, when, where, and how the eternal life of the soul is to be lived?

We have seen in the chapters on modern spiritualism and ancestor worship what the best answers yet given to these questions amount to. They are best because they give bodies to their souls just like those they had in earthlife, only of thinner stuff, and out of the same kind of stuff make a world just like this one for them so embodied to inhabit. Without a physical man and earth to copy from the constructors of the " land of the fathers", of the "land of the gods", of "the world of spirits", which certainly are the most credible and therefore best believed in of all the modes of immortality yet conceived of, might have produced nothing better than others have ; and even they, in respect to providing food for spirits assumed to be organized just like the hungry people of earth, have left their work sadly incomplete. Plainly a mode of immortality in the flesh and on the earth must have the same advantage over these that an original has over a copy. There are other theories, which furnish a subtle body to encase the soul, in order to its enjoying reward or suffering punishment, but such bodies, including those worn in the lands of the fathers and of the gods, are but temporary, and when finally they are shed the bare incorporeal supposition goes naked to its eternity. The Christian theory, according to which the soul leaves the body at death and afterwards returns to it again, is until such return peculiarly incredible, and gets still more so afterwards. The idea of terrestrial immortality is happily unincumbered with the idea of soul. To have assurance of it one need not be either a spiritualist or religionist, need not believe that what he recognizes as his soul, came down from the skies, or that it originated with his body, that it is an entity, or a mere result of the play of the forces of his animal organism. Whichever of these suppositions be true, or if none of them be, it is all the same to the expectant of a life to which death is neither the beginning nor the end. He knows that he now lives and knows how he lives, and sees no difficulty in remaining where he is and doing as he does. While the hypothesis of the immortality of the body is no more necessarily connected with religious belief than any other scientific hypothesis would be, that of the immortality of a detachable soul is so complicated with such belief that in order to know what is to become of him when he dies, a man has to find out which one of the many religions is true, a rather difficult task. If Hinduism be true, he is sure, in time, to get back to Brahman; if Christianity, he is to undergo his eternity either in a heaven where, for all we are told by those who claim to know, there is nothing to beguile his ennui for even one week, or in a hell, where, according to the same authority, the vast majority of us are to suffer in a way that if really believed in by any truly good man in the same way that he is able to believe in the ordinary occurrences of life, he would immediately die shrieking in sympathetic agony.

(It is true that some Christians say they have changed all that, and that there is to be no hell; but others say there is, and they are the wisest supporters of their faith; for if there is to be no hell for Christians there cannot be any heaven for them, the two resting on one and the same authority.) Thus incorporeal immortality, of itself quite hard enough to believe in, is made vastly more so by the added incredibilities of the religions which patronize it; by the incredible absurdities of their heavens and the incredible horrors of their hells. Corporeal immortality, on the other hand requires, in order to obtain belief, only the same kind of experimental knowledge and the same modes of reasoning all of us are accustomed to form our judgments on in everyday life; whether those avail to prove it is another thing.

To the reasons which have been given as having possibly led the Taoist to infer that the future transformations of man were to be in his present accustomed home, another may be added, which is that Nature's habit is to take no leaps. To go on with the task of perfecting man gradually and slowly would be in conformity to that habit; to kill him, in order to get his soul out of him and then send it, an unknown thing, to dwell in the unknown, would not; it would be a leap, and a leap in the dark.

CHAPTER XXX - CONCLUSION

But now let us put aside the hypothesis that yoga is a promise of terrestrial immortality, as we already have the hypothesis that it is the realization of it, and see if the problem it presents is made any easier by stripping it of these. If the wonderful and manifold facts attendant on the yoga movement (counting only such as are experimentally demonstrable), which have been set in array in the foregoing pages, mean neither coming immortality nor immortality to come, what do they mean ? At the least they mean the transformation of the practicer from an inferior into a superior man, which transformation consists in the acquisition of magical qualities and powers, the totality of which is nothing less than the whole body of magic. The data also show that magical quality and power are personal endowments, as much so as intellectual clearness or muscular energy, and as direct in their operation as these, that operation not being dependent on knowledge of any art or mystery, as some magicians have pretended, nor on the presence or aid of gods, spirits or demons, as others have, the operator doing all in virtue of his transformed nature. He has been created a magician by work done on his body which has improved it into a better instrument than it was for feeling, knowing and doing; and we do not know that anything else is needed to be done. He may fancy he has been exalted to be a god, and so may others, but he has only grown more perfect as a man. He has been taken up by the evolutionary movement and carried a stage further on his destined way, not by natural selection which calls death to its aid, and looks very much like chance, but by transformation, which comes with an augmented flow of life, and looks very much like design. That movement may be presumed to have taken hold on man as early as he was able to receive it, to have reached its fullest power as soon as the progress of civilization had secured the proper conditions for it, and to have ever been ready to enter into and abide with whoever would receive it.

I have said that the Siddhis, wonderful as they are, and able to support all religion and much philosophy, remained yet quantitatively scant, and so had been treated by the world at large, its churches and states, as unimportant, evil or unreal, which ill-reception and maltreatment has, by reacting on them, in turn become a cause working to render them more scanty still. But there have been many other causes, to wit, such as hinder all development that depends on the human intellect.

When the first distaff was wrapped with wool, and the first spindle twirled, the present spinning-jenny was begun. When first an ox was made to tread out corn, and the corn crushed between two stones, the threshing machine and new process flour-mill were effectively prophesied. But how long have these industrial inventions been in coming ! The world is young and growth is slow, and the development of magical methods, which could not certainly have begun any earlier than that of industrial ones, has had hindrances peculiar to itself. Religion has drunk up magic as a desert would a river. Heredity, which has so large a part in the other modes of evolution, plays little or no part in this, since celibacy is the prevailing condition of it, and its practice by celibates sterilizes. Thus the sphere and scope of the magical movement has been confined within very close limits, the practicer being in life cut off from all that concerns life, and in death dropping his body with all its painfully-won acquisitions. The fittest are in this way selected to die without progeny to inherit their fitness, and the least fit selected to survive in offspring who inherit their parents' unfitness. Painful and repulsive austerities, imparted by religion to yoga, have restricted its spread among the people, confining its sphere to the more fanatical members of society, excluding from it the open daylight of common sense, which would have aided it in improving its methods. But a still greater disadvantage has arisen from its recondite nature in the shape of laborious and tedious methods, erroneously supposed to be necessary.

Yoga being a movement of nature, from her ought to come all needed instruction in the practice of it; nor have these been withheld. The Rajah yogists, as we have seen, assert that simple concentration of the mind can set up in the body all the breathings and other movements in the intentional practice of which Hatha Yoga consists, and this assertion the American experiences prove to be true. Here, then, are revealed the requirements of nature respecting method, and, in the absence of other requirements in the same way revealed, the presumption is that all else is extraneous and needless. Thus nature has in an experimental way, whose meaning none need miss of, told man what to do in order to attain yoga. But then do those on whom she thus acts need instruction ? It would seem not, for she takes hold and does the practicing herself. The question here arises: Can all men, by simply stilling their minds by means of concentration, come to be thus acted on ? If there are any who cannot, then for such the experiences of those who can and are should serve as instruction, and the one class may be said to be in this way told how to attain to yoga, while the other may be said to be taken up and carried there. Probably if there be such difference in aptitude, it may depend on difference in the power of concentration, which all know to be very great. But inasmuch as all men have the power in some degree, it is possible that all may sooner or later attain. In so great a movement as the taking of the next step in the evolution of man, to trust to his contrivance or his volition, would be inconsistent with the habits of our mother, and this is another reason for inferring that all men are born with aptitude enough for her purpose. But in any case she must be supposed to have indicated in the movements in question the whole method of yoga practice needed as yet, and that no movement that will not come, whether to some men or all, as result of simple concentration should be esteemed good practice.

The improvement of method has hereto largely consisted in disencumbering it of painful, laborious and tedious austerities. It was to so disencumber Hindu Yoga that Sankaracharya wrote the commentary on the Vedanta before alluded to, or to give the words of his disciple : "To point out that the knowledge of Brahman is the only certain way of obtaining liberation, instead of the severe mortifications which mankind at present are incapable of performing". Old Taoism seems to have flung out as early as Lao-Tsee's time all that could be called "severe mortifications", if such ever had a place in its method of practice. John of the Cross, and his Carmelites of the bitterly severe unmitigated rite, heaped absurdities and cruelties on themselves, but soon after him came Molinos, with his "new method" in which penance had no place, and other religious performances very little, and got excellent results. In like manner with the acquisition of the siddhis the exercise of them has been much simplified. Paracelsus discarded all magical ritual and proclaimed that it was the imagination alone that did all. Gessner, who cured tens of thousands by true magic, thought it necessary to wear a scarlet cloak, a silken sash and a silver chain from which hung a fragment of the veritable cross, to pronounce the name of Jesus in exorcising disease and talk to the devil in Latin.

When Mesmer was told of all this he declared that the toggery and other accessories were useless and that the cures were performed by what he called "magnetic spiritual excitement", and proved it to the satisfaction of the Elector of Bavaria, But when Mesmer himself undertook to exhibit before a scientific committee the wonders of animal magnetism, he too thought it necessary to have his accessories in shape of a chemical apparatus equally useless with those of Gessner — that is to say, so thought until it was demonstrated that he could do just as good work without them; which caused the wiseacres of science, who witnessed both results, to decide that what could be done in two ways could be done in none, and that one of the greatest lights of his age was an impostor.

Since then mesmerism has been still more simplified, so that a glance of the eye, a few words or an unspoken thought will often produce as good effects as laborious manipulation of tedious duration formerly did. All which shows that magic can progress as well as other things; and it must be that soon or late it will fling off all remaining encumbrances and, freed from them, seek for and find as time goes on better and still better modes of practice until perfection of method is reached.

As objects of concentration the sensations have hitherto not been wholly neglected. The practicer is early encouraged by agreeable visitations through the channels of each sense in turn, and later becomes able at will to summon to their gratification lights, colors and forms, music, scents, tastes and touches of sweetness; and the witches' sleep and the lover's swoon prove that sensations of touch, at least, may be intensified to an extent that has no limit short of loss of consciousness in samadhi. What is thus proved true of one sense is inferentially true of the four others as well. Thus the possibility of improving method by simply intensifying sensation to a degree from which the practicer's attention will not be able to escape, and where perfect and absolute concentration will be assured, is great enough to permit the conjecture that by this way of the senses alone yoga methods may at some age in the future attain such perfection that all will be allured to practice them, and that too in the thorough way that has heretofore distinguished only two or three in a century of even the thorough-going Hindu sages, and the whole race of man become yogis.

www.ingramcontent.com/pod-product-compliance
Lightning Source LLC
Chambersburg PA
CBHW071018280326
41935CB00011B/1403